Crystal Harmony
Healing properties of crystals & how to use them to harmonise your life

By Debra Cushing BHSc Nat

Crystal Harmony: Healing properties of crystals & how to use them to harmonise your life
A self-published title
Debra Cushing
PO Box 5560
Alexandra Hills Qld 4161
Australia
deb@redraspberrynaturopathics.com.au
www.redraspberrynaturopathics.com.au

First Published in 2016
Copyright text © Debra Cushing
Copyright photographs © Debra Cushing
Cover design © Debra Cushing

All rights reserved. This book or any portion thereof may not be reproduced or used in any manner whatsoever without the express written permission of the publisher except for the use of brief quotations in a book review.

Printed by IngramSpark

ISBN 978-0-9954154-0-9

The author of this book does not dispense medical advice or prescribe the use of any technique as a form of treatment for physical or medical problems without the advice of a health care professional, either directly or indirectly. The intent of the author is only to offer information of a general nature to help in the quest for emotional and spiritual wellbeing. The author assumes no responsibility for any information used by the reader.

Dedicated to my beautiful children, Ryan and Sabrina, who love playing with crystals as much as I do.

Special thanks to my husband, Nigel, who supported and accepted my obsession with crystals. Thanks to my BFF Christina, who encouraged me to put my knowledge and love of crystals into a book.

Contents

Introduction	7
How Crystals Work	8
How to Choose Your Crystals	10
Cleansing and Energising Crystals	11
Programming	15
Getting to know your crystal	17
Types of Crystals	18
Fake Crystals – What to look out for	20
Crystal Systems – Basic Shape and Geometric forms	22
Traditional Colour Meanings	23
Amethyst	26
Argonite (Blue)	28
Black Tourmaline	30
Carnelian	33
Celestite	34
Citrine	37
Clear Quartz	38
Fluorite	40
Green Aventurine	42
Hematite	43
Herkimer Diamond	44
Honey (Golden) Calcite	45
Iolite	46
Kyanite	48
Labradorite	51
Lapis Lazuli	52
Lepidolite	53
Malachite	54
Moldavite	55

Moonstone	57
Obsidian	58
Phantom Quartz	60
Red Jasper	61
Rose Quartz	62
Selenite	65
Smokey Quartz	67
Sodalite	68
Tiger Eye	70
Yellow Jade	72
Grids	74
Messages from the crystals	76
Environment – windows, doorways, beds, TV's, electrical equipment, garden	77
Gem Waters / Essences	79
Pendants / Jewelery	80
Healing / Chakra Balancing	81
Pendulum	85
Correspondences	86
Bibliography	91

Introduction

This book is the results of over 20 years collecting, researching and working with crystals. I have been extremely blessed over the years when it comes to crystals – I have some extraordinary specimens, I have even been lucky enough to visit the Herkimer Diamond mine in Herkimer, New York, before the mine closed – I was even luckier to be able to bring some Herkimer matrix's back to Australia. For many years I have worked with crystals for personal use, as a crystal healer, in 2009 I also developed a range of 13 crystal essences. I found that people would seek me out to identify a crystal for them or to ask questions about particular crystals or on how they can be used. I knew that even after completing a Bachelor of Health Science I still wanted to include my love of crystals in my work. This was the initial inspiration to hold crystal workshops, so participants could experience the crystals in my collection, to ask questions and for me to pass on information. So after many months sitting at the computer doing more research and getting all the information out of my head and onto the page in order to teach an introductory crystal workshop, I found I had so much information. I get so passionate talking about crystals and can go on for hours, literally, and yet after 8hrs I still didn't get through all the information for the introductory workshop. With 2 small children I was finding it hard to hold workshops, so the next best thing was to turn the workshop manual into a book – here it is!

Crystals have many different colours, crystalline structures, shapes, sizes and chemical compositions which contribute to their many meanings and purposes. The healing qualities of each crystal come from thousands of years use and anecdotal evidence. Then there is the specific quality each individual crystal has on each individual person. Two people can hold the same piece and get 2 different feelings from it, this is what that person needs at that moment from that particular crystal. The crystal information in this book is from both ancient knowledge and channeled information.

How Crystals Work

In order for crystals to be more effective and 'work', they need to be actively worked with – to be held and touched. Crystals have a relatively small electromagnetic field (EMF) whilst sitting there looking pretty, but when held, heat and friction excite the electrons and molecules (this is the essence of nature) which increases their EMF.

This can be seen by triboluminescence[1] and piezoelectric[2] crystals such as quartz and tourmaline, which is why they are used in watches and hair straighteners. When heated, tourmaline and quartz develop electrical charges on their opposing faces – one side positive ions the other negative ions. This electrical polarity has been beneficial in the development of hair straighteners as the negative ions help to reduce frizz. The EMF can also be measured / seen by the use of divining rods.

The chemical composition is also of importance as each chemical element has its own vibrational frequency. This is of use especially in the body – to bring it back into alignment to the right frequency. Smoky Quartz and Lepidolite both contain lithium in their chemical composition; both crystals are beneficial for use in depression as they both help to retune the lithium frequency in the body. Lithium is sometimes used in medical science to treat biopolar disorder and depression.

When we come into contact with the crystals EMF it has an effect on the energetic body. The electromagnetic field can influence energy flow through the meridians; activate and balance the chakra; stimulate electrical nerve impulses; activate and regulate hormonal glands; cells, tissue and organ metabolism.

---

1 **Triboluminescence** - the emission of light from a substance caused by rubbing, scratching or similar frictional contact.
2 **Piezoelectric** - the ability of certain materials to generate an electric charge in response to applied mechanical stress

Moh's Scale of Hardness

The scale of hardness/softness of a mineral was developed by German scientist Friedrich Mohs. Minerals higher on the scale will be able to scratch minerals lower and minerals lower on the scale can be scratched by those above it and they can also disintegrate in water.

1. Talc – can be scratch by fingernail
2. Gypsum – can be scratched by fingernail
3. Calcite – can be scratched by a copper coin
4. Fluorite – can be scratched by a knife
5. Apatite – can just be scratched by a knife
6. Feldspar – can be scratched by a steel file
7. Quartz – can scratch glass
8. Topaz – can scratch quartz
9. Corundum – can scratch topaz
10. Diamond – hardest known natural mineral

How to Choose Your Crystals

We do not own crystals, we are their temporary custodian – whether you paid for the piece, it was given to you or whether it was found. This is why we sometimes 'lose' them – it was time the crystal moved on to a new custodian. If you listen, they will speak to you and they will let you know when it's time to move on.

Size, colour and shape have no bearing when it comes to which stone you should work with. If you ask a child why those chose a particular stone, they are more likely to answer "because I like the way it feels".

When choosing a stone, whether in nature or in a shop, pick up the first one that attracts you. Hold it in your receptive hand[3] and sense how it feels – hot, cold, comforting, vibrating, slimy. If you don't feel comfortable with the stone don't buy it. If it feels very negative or slimy to you, try the next one. Keep trying until you feel one that it is right for you.

Sometimes a crystal will choose you! If a crystal cuts you, it is trying to get your attention. It may be a sign that you need to work with that crystal; or it is infusing some of its energies with you. If the crystal is for sale, the crystal Deva is not taking any chances of not getting your attention. If you already own the crystal and it cuts you, you may not even feel the cut at the time, it is the melding and forging of energies to have a deeper connection.

---

3 **Receptive hand** – regardless if you are left or right handed, the receptive hand is on your left. The reason behind this is the left hand is closest to the heart, the left side of the body is associated with spirituality, psychic ability, love and wisdom. The right side is associated with power, healing, protection, courage and self-confidence, making your right hand your projective hand.

Cleansing and Energising Crystals

Before the crystals come to us, they have picked up many energies. When buying from a shop – how many people of touched them before we take them home? How has their energy been effected by the mining process? The acid wash cleaning process? The tumbling process? The dyeing / lacquering process (if they have been dyed or lacquered)? These will all affect the energetic strength of the crystal. So first thing you need to do before you do any work with a new crystals is to cleanse and energise them. The only exception to this is if you find a piece in nature; but before you pick it up to take it home, you need to ask the crystals permission. If the answer is no, leave it where it is. Also be aware of any local government licenses and permission you may need (fossiking and/or land owner).

Different techniques for cleansing:
Under running water / ocean
- Best for natural water – in a stream, ocean or out whilst raining – crystals will only need 2-3 minutes in a rainstorm to be cleansed and energized.
- Filtered tap water and as a last resort normal tap water.
- I always recite the following affirmation when using running water: "I ask the universe to cleanse this crystal with love and respect and to wash away all negativities. Blessed Be"

Tip: This technique should not to be used on any water soluble crystals such as Selenite or crystals with a Mohs hardness under 4.

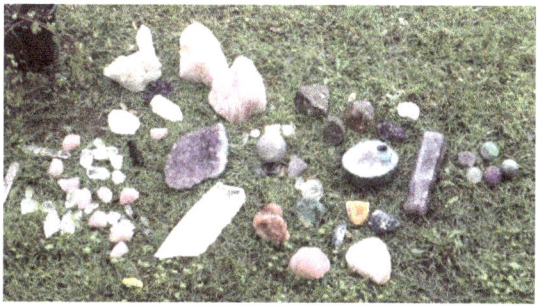

Sound
Tibetan bells or symbols, tuning forks, crystal bowls, drumming or chanting helps to clear unwanted vibrations. Sound can help to the crystal return to its original oscillating frequency especially after its mining and initial processing.

Sun / moon
Leave crystal in sunlight and moonlight for 24hours.
The full moon is a good time, as the moon rises at the same time the sun sets so there is a continuous flow of energy.

Tip: some crystals will fade if left in the sun for a full day – quartz family

Nature - Burying in the ground
Bury and leave crystal in the ground for 1-2weeks or a full moon cycle (28 days). Bury at full moon and unearth at new moon.

Tip: remember where you buried it!!!! (sometimes it is beneficial to put it in a plant pot).

Put the crystal in a pot of herbs associated with general healing – lavender, sage or rosemary, for 24 hours.

Broken crystals can also be buried to help 'heal' their energy flow, however they do need a long time in the ground (months to years)
- A note about crystals that break.
  Common causes: physical impact (dropped), sudden temperature changes (thermal shock), energetic impact (high oscillating frequencies).

  Broken crystals can still be used - their energy hasn't diminished. Crystals that have shattered can still be used also – the dust and small particles can be placed in a garden bed to assist in the growing of plants. As there is a link between fragments of the one piece, it widens the energetic field in which it is working. Imagine if a piece of black tourmaline broke into 4 pieces and you used it in a protection grid around your house – it would be very strong as all pieces have that extra link of being from the one whole.
  Don't despair, they can break for a number of reasons – if you no

longer need the benefit of the crystal to have or to wear (jewelery / pendants). The crystal may have fulfilled its purpose with you, so may break / shatter or many become lost. Sometimes the crystal may break in order for you to pass a piece of it onto someone else.

Fire – candle flame
Pass the crystal through the flame of a candle 3 times.

Tip: Some crystal change colour when heated (amethyst).

Placing on cluster
Clusters are very purifying and can be used to cleanse all other crystals. Place crystal on a cluster for 24hrs.

Tip: If using a cluster for cleansing other crystals, the cluster will need to be cleansed approximately once per week.

Incense/smudging
Circle the crystal in the smoke form sage, sandalwood, frankincense or myrrh incense or a smudge stick.

Reiki
If you have been attuned to Reiki, you can use the Sei He Ki symbol to cleanse the crystals. Cho Ku Rei can also be used to energise them.

Rice
Rice absorbs energy. Place crystal in rice for 24hrs, then dispose of the rice.

Pendulum
Hold clear quartz pendulum over the crystal (delicate shades are best cleansed with an amethyst or rose quartz pendulum), pass the pendulum over the crystal nine times with slow anti-clockwise circles to remove negativity.
Dip the pendulum into a bowl of cold water nine times and shake it dry (be aware of thermal shock). Finally, move the pendulum nine times clockwise over the crystal to empower it.

Sprays – cleansing
Clearing and cleansing sprays
Blessed water
Full moon water
Sun water
Herbal infusion sprays – lavender, rosemary, sage

Other
Lightning, meteor showers, rainbows, cold

The cold makes it difficult to hold onto vibrations – be aware that extreme temperature changes may crack the crystal.
Example: Icelandic Spar – if it was mined in Iceland its natural environment is a cold climate and cleanses well in the cold or when surrounded by ice. Moldavite is formed when a meteorite impacted the earth, so cleansing and engerising it during a meteor shower is really powerful.

Tip: remember to take the Elemental qualities of the crystal into consideration – using water to cleanse a fire crystal may dampen its energy – to combat this, remember to energize using a fire element

Energising
Other ways to energise crystals not listed under cleansing, include:
- Using the Planet associated with the crystal, crystals can be placed outside on the days associated with that planet.
- Star power – determine zodiac constellation that sun, moon and planets occupy.
- Elemental power – Earth, Air, Fire, Water.
- Sprays – Full moon, new moon, sun waters (water that has been set out in a bowl under the full moon, new moon or in the sun to absorb its vibrational energy).

Programming

Just about every book you pick up on crystals or website you visit, always has a section on programming crystals. I don't nor have I ever programmed a crystal and here's my thoughts on it.

Why I don't program....

When I was first introduced to crystals I had never read a book on them and it was long before the use of the internet. I found out what their basic use was from the 'tag' on the piece of jewelry an also developed a relationship with the crystals simply by sitting with and 'listening' to the tumbled pieces I had. I felt their spirit and recognized them as 'other beings'. I treated them with respect and treated them as I like to be treated. I hate to be told what to do, so why would the crystals be any different. That is not to say you cannot 'ask' them to help you in your work. I have found that they (as well as myself) give more when asked to help and are not told to do so. Then the first books I read on crystals were by DJ Conway and Scott Cunningham in the 90's, neither of these authors mentioned programming crystals.

The crystals know why they are here and what their energy is for, who are we to change their purpose, why not nurture their strengths and ask to harness that energy. If we listen they will tell us.

The more you work with your crystals, you get to know them and they get to know you, the more time you spend with them the more effective the working relationship will be. Once connected with the crystals deva/spirit/guardian it's a sign of respect to ask for their help not tell them. When I do a crystal healing I have several crystal points that I choose from, I will ask the guardians of those crystals which one wishes to assist in the energy healing session for that person.

We do not OWN crystals, we are only their temporary custodian. This is why we sometimes 'lose' them – it was time to go to a new custodian. If you listen, they will speak to you and they will let you know when it's time to move on.

Some people charge exuberant prices for crystals that have been 'charged', 'energised', 'programmed' or 'attuned' for you or by a certain person. No thanks, that's not for me. Not only are you trusting that that person had pure intentions when doing it, but the 'attunement' is only very short term – it's not permanent – which is why when setting crystal grids you need to keep activating it at regular intervals (more on that later). You will find that if you get to know your crystal yourself and work with it, you will have a deeper connection and a more powerful personal effect.

Getting to know your crystal

Sit with your crystal for 5-10 minutes to get to know the feel of it.
Make sure you a sitting in a comfortable seat. Have the crystal sitting on a table or on the floor in front of you. Have it close enough so that you can gaze at it without straining your eyes.
Sit with your eyes closed and take a couple of deep breaths to centre yourself. Be aware of how you are feeling. Take note of your emotional state; your thoughts; mood. Is your mind active or quiet? Do you keep focusing on a certain issue?
Now tune into your body and be aware of how it feels. Are there any areas of discomfort or tension? or do you feel some other sensation?
Now that you know how you are feeling its time to turn your attention to the crystal. Start by simply gazing at your chosen crystal for a minute or two.
Pick up the crystal and take a couple of deep breaths as you assimilate with the crystal. Then examine it closely from all angles.
After a minute or so, hold the crystal between your hands and close your eyes. Once again scan your body, mind and emotions, do you notice any differences, however slight?
Continue to hold your crystal and breathe deeply for another couple of minutes and take notice of any changes that are occurring or any messages you may receive.

Types of Crystals

Wands

Crystal wands come in many different shapes and sizes. They can be short or long, the body may be faceted or cylindrical and smooth. They can have a terminated point at one end and rounded at the other. They can be rounded at both ends or they can be double terminated with points at both ends. Some wands are wider at one end and tapered at the other. Wands come in many varieties of crystals, most have been cut, shaped and polished. However, rough natural pointed crystals, such as quartz, can also be used as a healing wand.

Wands are used to gather and focus energy through their points. The elongated, cylindrical shape enables the crystal to direct its healing energy in a straight line. Using a crystal wand in reflexology and massage can assist in healing, at both a physical and deep energetic level. Using your own energy can drain you making you feel fatigued, weak and depleted and in need of healing yourself, so it is important to allow universal healing energy to flow in through your crown chakra, down your arm to the hand holding the wand, then into the wand where it is amplified and passed into the patient.

Tip: I have used a rose quartz massage wand on a red, lumpy scar, which had been there for a couple of years. The next day, after one healing session, the scar was no longer lumpy and it was barely noticable – it had changed colour overnight to very pale pink/skin colour.

Terminated and double terminated

Energy flows in the direction of the point. Single terminated points (usually pointed down) direct the energy flow down to the ground, this can be grounding, soothing, calming and energerising, be mindful that it does not drain you. When it is pointed up it strengthens the spirit and is uplifting – good for meditation and contemplation, however be careful you don't become too light headed or unfocused. Double terminated points allow for energy flow in both directions.

Geodes
Geodes are especially powerful for cleansing, purifying and balancing energy in a room.

Clusters
Clusters are usually sections of geodes. They help balance a rooms energy and are useful for cleansing other crystals.

Spheres
Scrying, massage. All crystal spheres operate through your crown chakra.

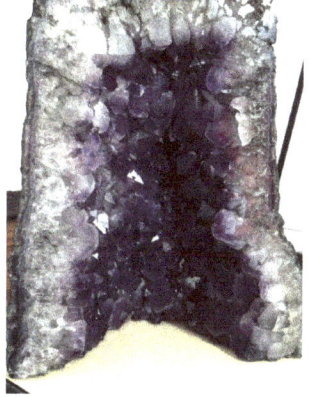

Tumbled/ chips
Useful for grids, medicine[4] or mojo[5] bags and constructing barriers. Some tumbled stones may be lacquered due to fibres that may be harmful and also to increase shine.

Natural Crystals
Crystals in their rough or raw state – some may be lacquered due to fibres that may be harmful.

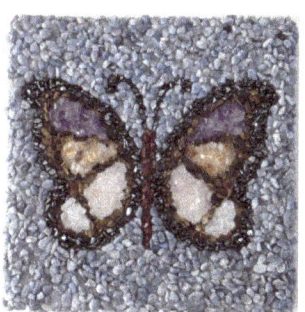

Cabochon
A crystal with flat back surface, mostly used in jewellery.

Faceted Stones
Gem quality crystals used in jewellery.

---

4 **Medicine bag**: pouch used for the intent of healing, can include crystals & herbs
5 **Mojo bag**: pouch used for holding ingredients of a spell or magickal working

Fake Crystals – What to look out for

Just about all citrine on the market is heat treated amethyst - I don't see this as too much of an issue for a couple of reasons:
1. They both have the chemical composition of silicon dioxide,
2. Amethyst and citrine have the same crystalline structure (after all natural citrine was amethyst that was heated by Mother Earth),
3. Both heat treated amethyst and citrine are a yellow/ orange colour.

Obsidian - is volcanic glass - made by a volcano (if it wasn't made by a volcano it's just glass) - it only comes in black (mahogany, rainbow and snowflake obsidian is black obsidian with inclusions). Geologist have yet to confirm any naturally occurring blue or green obsidian which is supposedly from Mount St Helen's. It definitely doesn't come in purple - these are just coloured glass.

I've recently come across 'cal-silica' or 'rainbow cal-silica'. These are actually dried layers of car paint and plastic. Sometimes it also contains ground up calcite in it!

Irradiated Crystals
These are real crystals that have been irradiated to enhance and deepen colours and some even change colour. Are these safe? well they can hold onto the radiation, so I wouldnt be carrying it around on me. The natural crystals that mother earth radiated slowly over a long period of time is not radioactive. The colours fade pretty quick on radiated crystals when put in sun, naturally radiated ones takes a lot longer to fade.

Crystals that are most commonly irradiated:
- deep colour kunzite
- very deep pink/red tourmaline
- deep colour topaz
- coloured diamonds
- very dark (almost black) smoky quartz

Turquoise is one of the most common crystals that is faked, it usually dyed howlite or magnesite. The dyed turquoise does not have colour all the way through, so if you scratch it with a knife and see white, it's a fake.

Look at the scratch under magnification, if the edge is tattered - its real, if its smooth - its fake. Real turquoise will also burn if you put the tip of a hot needle on it, fake turquoise will melt. You can also use a black light to see if it has been reconstituted - ground up turquoise that has had resin added to it to shape it - the resin with glow under the black light. Real Turquoise has a triclinic crystal system whereas howlite is monoclinic and magnesite is hexagonal.

You can tell if your quartz and agates have been dyed as the dye can collect in the cracks (they are now selling 'crackled quartz' which is all dyed) most of those bright coloured agates are actually dyed.

Bizmuth - whilst it is an element on the periodic table, the pretty rainbow bizmuth crystals in the shops are made in a lab. Natural bizmuth is a dull grey colour.

Goldstone (aka aventurine glass) - it is manmade molten copper and glass - it looks awesome, but it's not a real crystal.

Opalite (sometimes labeled as moonstone) is manmade glass or sometimes even plastic

Unfortunately some shops and people who sell crystals may not be aware that what they are selling is not real (fake) or irradiated, as they believe what their wholesaler says the crystal is and they are selling it because it looks pretty. I have been a crystal junkie (lol) for over 20 years and it's only been in the last 6-7 years I have become more aware of the fakes as there a lot more on the market. Anything with a trademark name is either fake or a combination stone that someone decided to rename and trademark in order to charge more money for it, look closely at anything with a fruit name (I'm not saying these are all fake, but some definitely are, some are just using a more appealing name for it)

Crystal Systems – Basic Shape and Geometric Forms

The outer form of the crystal will not necessarily reflect its inner structure (however it does affect how energy flows through it)

Hexagonal
Created from hexagons, forming a 3d shape. Highly energetic, useful for energy balancing and exploring specific issues.

Cubic
Created from squares with axis at right angles to each other. Extremely stabilizing and grounding, useful for structure and reorganization.

Tip: This is the only crystal form that does not bend light rays as they pass through it.

Trigonal
Created from triangles. Radiate energy and are invigorating and protective, rebalancing the biomagnetic sheath.

Tetragonal
Created from rectangles with long and short axis at right angles. Absorb and transform energy and are excellent balancers and resolvers.

Orthorhombic
Created from rhomboids. Have unequal axises that encompass energy and are useful cleansers and clearers.

Triclinic
Created from trapeziums. Asymmetric triclinic crystals integrate energy and opposites and assist in exploring other dimensions.

Monoclinic
Created from parallelograms. Useful for purification and perception.

Amorphous
Lacks an inner structure. Allows energy to pass through freely and act rapidly and may be a catalyst for growth.

Traditional Colour Meanings

Red Crystals
Increase your power, excitement, passion, courage and physical energy. Communication.

Pink Crystals
Kindness, love and compassion for yourself and others.

Orange Crystals
Enhance creativity, self-esteem and confidence.

Yellow Crystals
Encourages optimism and alertness, positive attitude and assists self-expression

Green Crystals
Promotes harmony, balance and soothes emotions. Aids growth, renewal and healing

Blue Crystals
Relaxing and restful, Calms the mind, soothes and cools the physical body.

Purple Crystals
Enhances spiritual knowledge and developing intuition

Black Crystals
Powerful protectors, helps transmute negative energy and stress. Self Analysis of thoughts.

Brown Crystals
Grounding, practicality, safety.

White or Clear Crystals
Promotes new beginnings, peace and tranquility, clarity of purpose, spiritual insights. Increases the flow of life force

The Crystals

Amethyst

Crystal System: Trigonal
Astrological: Pisces, Virgo, Aquarius, Capricorn
Chakra: Third Eye, Crown
Element: Air and Water
Planet: Jupiter, Neptune
Hardness: 7
Composition: SiO_2 – Silicon Dioxide with Iron
Common Sources: Worldwide

Healing
- Purification and healing
- Balancing spiritual and physical
- Reduces negativity
- Cleanses the blood
- Calms the mind, inner peace and strength
- Cleanses/purifies
- Understanding dreams
- Creativity
- Align emotions
- Strengthens immunity
- Meditation
- Aids in falling asleep – reduces nightmares and insomnia
- Helps with physical pain, headaches, migraines
- Aids negotiations, decision-making, wealth, business success
- Assists moving forward in life, coping with responsibility and change
- Relieves stress and tension

Magical
- Develops psychic ability
- Facilitates connection to Guides and Angels
- Meditation and intuition, inspiration, channeling
- Brings about change

- Protection
- Transformation
- Spiritual development

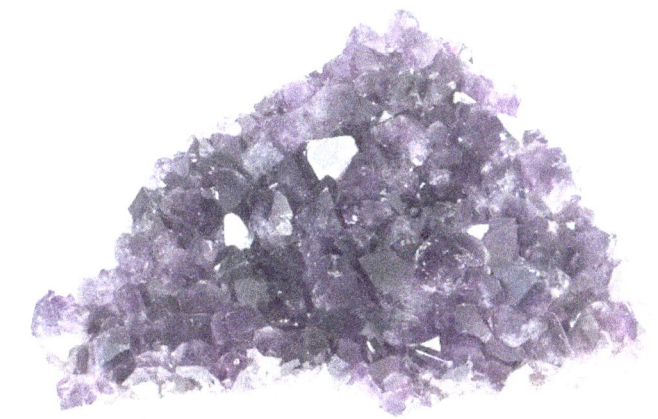

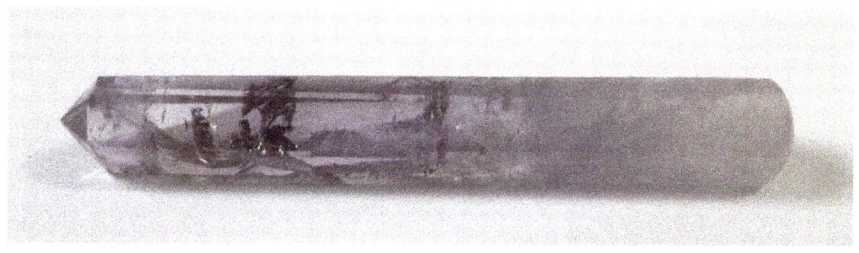

Argonite (Blue)

Crystal System: Orthorhombic
Astrological: Capricorn
Chakra: Third Eye, Throat, Heart
Element: Earth
Planet: Earth
Hardness: 3.5-4
Composition: $CaCo_3$ – Calcium carbonate with impurities
Common Sources: UK, Spain, USA, Morocco

Healing
- Increases optimism
- Brings about new ideas and opportunities to grow
- Purifies and aligns subtle bodies with the physical
- Balances yin-yang
- Calms over-sensitivities
- Stops nightmares and night terrors in children
- Diffuses anger, stress, impatience and harsh words
- Good for problem-solving
- Communication – being able to speak up, aiding confidence in being able to speak the truth, to get across what you need to say.

Magical
- Heightens and grounds spiritual communication
- Earth healer and grounding
- Excellent for Goddess and outdoor rituals
- Transforms geopathic stress and ley line blockages
- Assists in recognizing root cause of problems and gently takes back to childhood and beyond to heal

♦ Unveiling the third eye and releasing the brain of fogginess and dizziness

♦ Out of the mundane – crossing dimensions, past life connections of simpler times, connecting to nature and unplugging from technology.

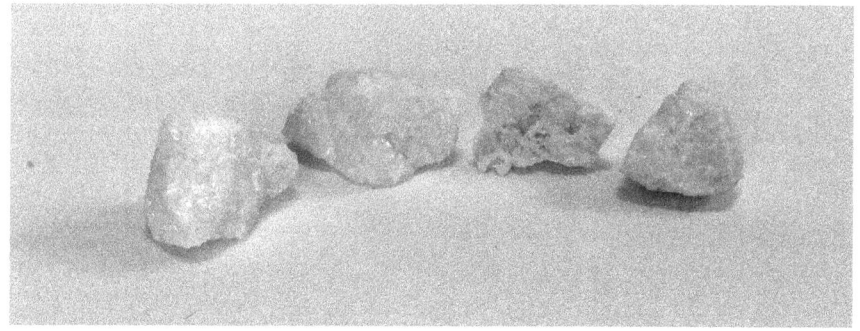

Black Tourmaline

Crystal System: Trigonal
Astrological: Libra
Chakra: Root
Element: Earth
Planet: Pluto
Hardness: 7
Composition: Complex borosilicate
Common sources: Sri Lanka, Africa, Australia, USA, Brazil, Afghanistan, Madagascar, Italy, Germany,

Healing
- Helps with flexibility, concentration, self discipline, independent thinking, courage, individuality, self-confidence and understanding abstract ideas
- Changes and release internal negativity
- Truth / honesty
- Stability in change
- Good for fear, obstruction, victim mentality, worrying what others think
- Yin/yang balance
- Release/letting go
- Travel
- Assists in labour/child birth – letting go

Magical
- Re-birthing
- Strengthens astral travel
- Protective shield – deflects physical and psychic negative energies Achievement
- Wards off fear and negativity,
- Anchor higher vibrations of light into physical body
- Processing information from past lives
- Inner wisdom

- ♦ Strengthens astral travel
- ♦ Can cause vibrations or events to slow down so you can assess things better
- ♦ Grounding

Sometimes found as a rod in quartz – energy enhancement, healing cellular memory (multidimensional), very effective in neutralizing psychic attack. Integrates the shadow into whole person and to move beyond duality
"If you handle your pieces of tourmaline often, they become extremely sensitive to your vibrations and rapidly respond to whatever you are doing." (DJ Conway p242)

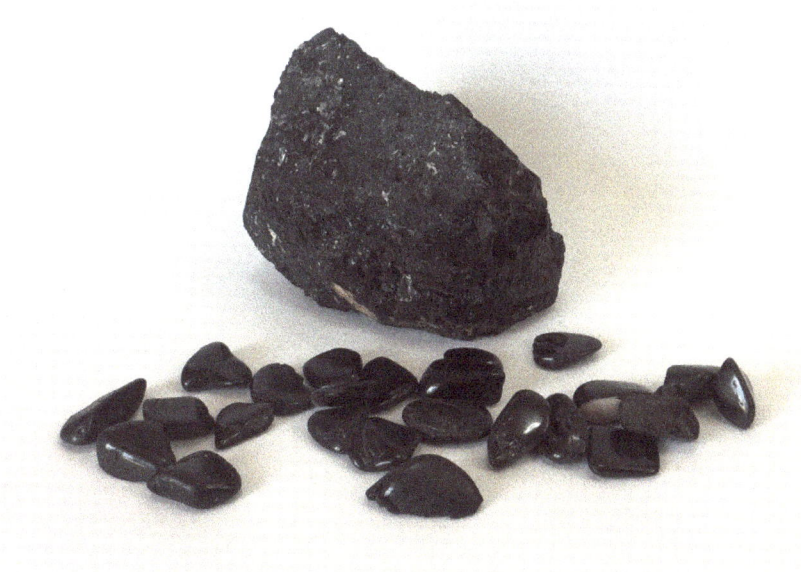

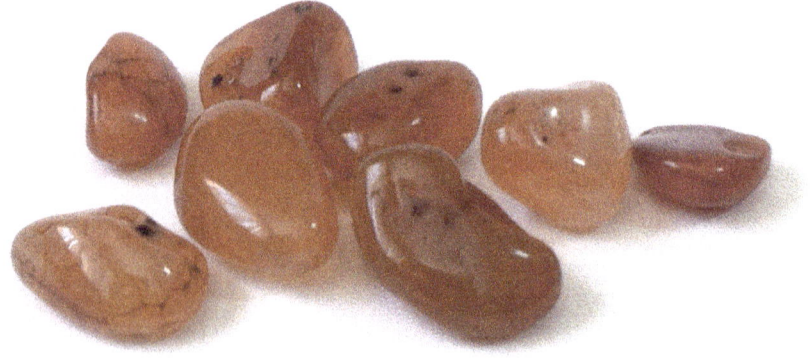

Carnelian

Crystal System: Trigonal
Astrological: Taurus, Cancer, Leo, Scorpio
Chakra: Root, Sacral
Element: Fire
Planet: Sun
Hardness: 7
Composition: SiO_2 + (Fe, O, OH) Silicon dioxide with impurities
Common Sources: Brazil, Russia, India, Australia, Madagascar, South Africa, Uruguay, USA, UK, Peru, Iceland

Healing
- Calms emotions – anger, jealousy and envy
- Restores vitality
- Acceptance of cycle of life
- Removes fear of death
- Assists positive life choices
- Overcome the fear of public speaking
- Increases sense of self-worth
- Helps to trust yourself and your perceptions.
- Overcoming negative conditioning.
- Stimulates concentration and memory

Magical
- Cleanses other stones
- Abundance – motivates success in business.
- Used in rituals to speed manifestation
- Aids understanding inner self
- Excellent for career success
- Wear on right hand to protect from cording
- Wear in a ring on left hand to remember astral travel or when checking into past lives
- Prevents others from reading your thoughts or dark forces from influencing the mind

Celestite

Crystal System: Orthorhombic
Astrological: Gemini
Chakra: Throat, Third Eye, Crown, Soul Star
Element: Water, Air
Planet: Venus, Neptune, Jupiter
Hardness: 3-3.5
Composition: $SrSO_4$ – Strontium Sulfate
Common Sources: UK, Egypt, Madagascar, Libya, Poland, Peru

Healing
- Aids calmness and serenity
- Purity of the heart
- Harmonises the environment
- Assists dysfunctional relationships: healing and release of emotional abuse
- Enhances respectful love, harmony and peace
- Enhances natural abilities
- Calming and balancing of fiery emotions and instinct
- Assists in public speaking and creative expression - especially in front of large crowds
- Releasing neck pain associated with carrying the weight of the world on shoulders

Magical
- Brings divine energy into environment
- Assists with connecting to Guides, Guardian Angels and Divine Angels
- Essential for dream recall and astral travel
- Heals the Aura
- Enhances metaphysical and spiritual development
- Trust in the wisdom of the divine and the universe
- Protects from lower vibrational energies

♦ Healing DNA structures and cellular memory to reconnect to our angelic selves
♦ Higher vibrational consciousness

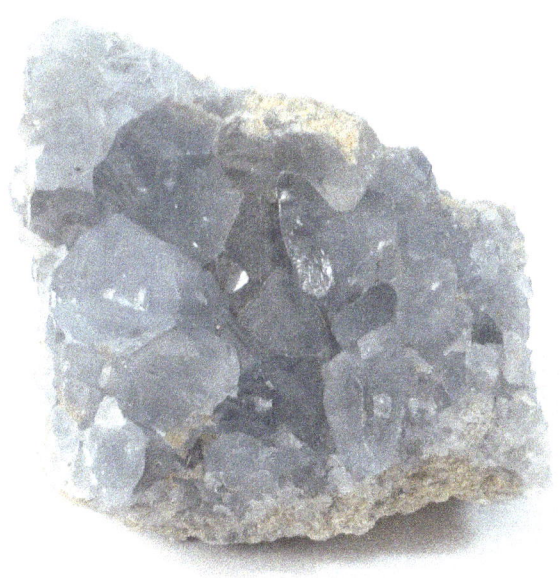

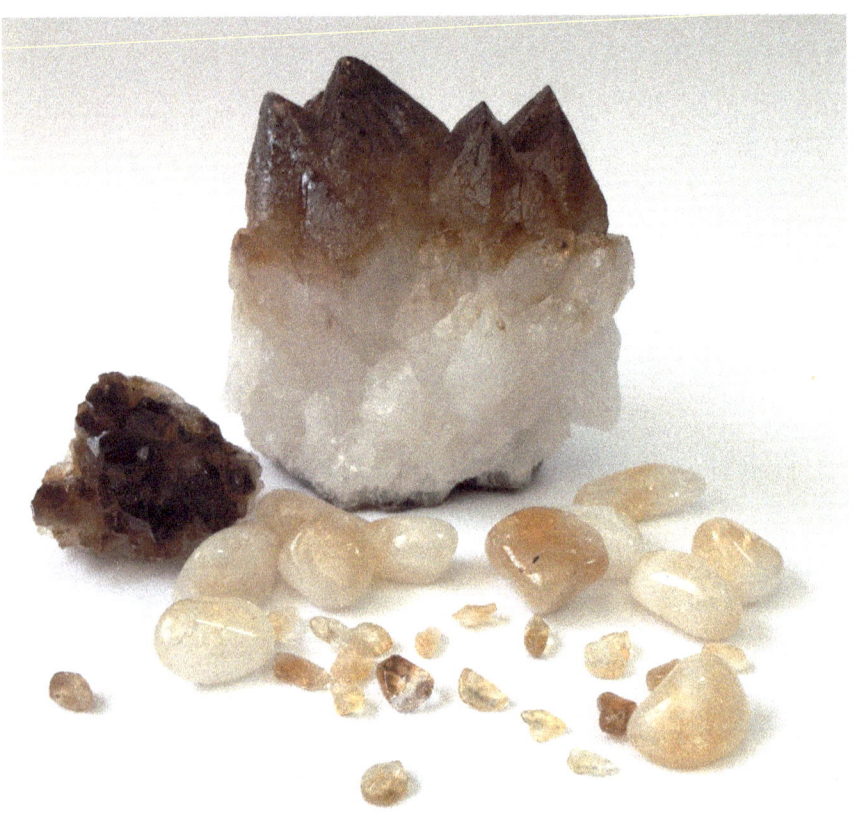

*unfortunately most citrine on the market is actually heat treated amethyst

Citrine

Crystal System: Trigonal
Astrological: Scorpio
Chakra: Solar Plexus
Element: Fire
Planet: Sun
Hardness: 7
Composition: SiO2 – Silicon Dioxide
Common sources: UK, USA, Brazil, France, Madagascar, Russia,

Healing
- Transforms emotional fears
- Clarity of thought
- Increases motivation
- Creative energy
- Environmental toxins
- Increases optimism
- Personal power
- Raises self-esteem, self-love
- Aids decision making, learning, teaching, studying, creativity, problem solving, flexibility
- Getting rid of emotional toxins. Eliminate self-destructive tendencies
- Helps anger and yin/yang balance

Magical
- Protect aura – healing and clearing Use to align with higher self.
- Manifestation
- "Money stone' - Abundance, attracts prosperity, good for business success
- New beginnings

Clear Quartz

Crystal System: Hexagonal
Astrological: All
Chakra: All, Crown
Element: Fire and Water – Storm
Planet: Sun and Moon
Hardness: 7
Composition: SiO_2 – Silicon Dioxide
Common sources: USA, Brazil, China, Madagascar, Russia, South Africa, Tibet

Healing
- All-purpose healer
- Emotional balancer
- Stimulates thinking processes
- Stimulates brain function
- Physical healing
- Stamina
- Travel
- Wellbeing enhancer
- Improves quality of life
- Increases happiness
- Affinity for pineal and pituitary glands

Magical
- Channels any energy - helps any condition
- Aids meditation
- Relieves negativity
- Receives, activates, transmits and amplifies energy
- Meditation – enhances communication with higher self, spirit guides, interdimensional entities
- Enhances psychic powers
- Amplifies energy
- Energizes all levels of consciousness

- Repels and destroys negative energies and vibrations
- Helps heal diabetes, ear infections, hearing and balance, heart health, malaise, obesity, pain, tinnitus

Why Quartz??? Our cells and body each have their own EMF, so does mother earth. Our cells EMF is maintained by silica (the human body holds approx 7g of Silica) – spending as little as 5mins in meditation with crystals (quartz) can help transmute the energy entering your EMF. Quartz helps to realign the body's own EMF

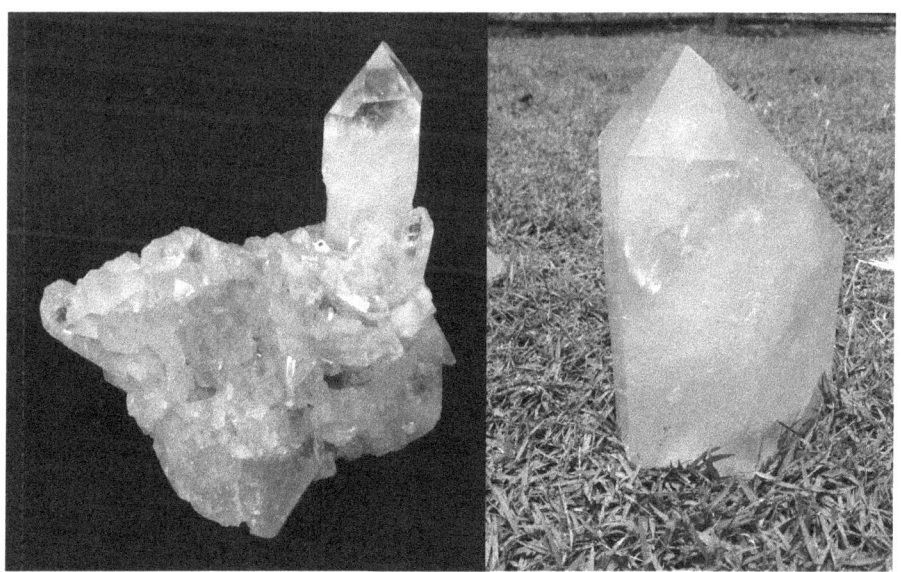

Fluorite

Crystal System: Cubic
Astrological: Pisces, Capricorn
Chakra: All
Element: Wind
Planet: Neptune
Hardness: 4
Composition: $CaFl_2$ – Calcium Fluoride
Common Sources: Brazil, England, Mexico, Canada, Australia, Germany, Norway, China, Peru, USA

Healing
- Helps regulate pain, inflammation, balance, co-ordination, psychosomatic disease, nerve related pain
- Antiviral - reducing side effects from infections, DNA damage, shingles
- Health of stomach, intestines and colon. Helps colitis, heartburn, nausea and sore throat, blood vessels and spleen
- Dealing with complex issues
- Letting Go/Releasing
- Reduces radiation
- Helps absorb nutrients
- Excellent for study or work areas – focus, concentration, clarity and memory

Magical
- Ground excessive energy – emotional, mental and nervous
- Cleansing the aura
- Clears negativity from room
- Psychic protections - rids and repels cording
- Aids channeling and Intuition
- Akashic records – past lives
- Excellent for concentration and meditation – enhances understanding and perceptiveness

- Inter-dimensional communication
- Understanding

It helps us to 'walk our talk', if you are not on your correct path it helps to bring us back onto our path

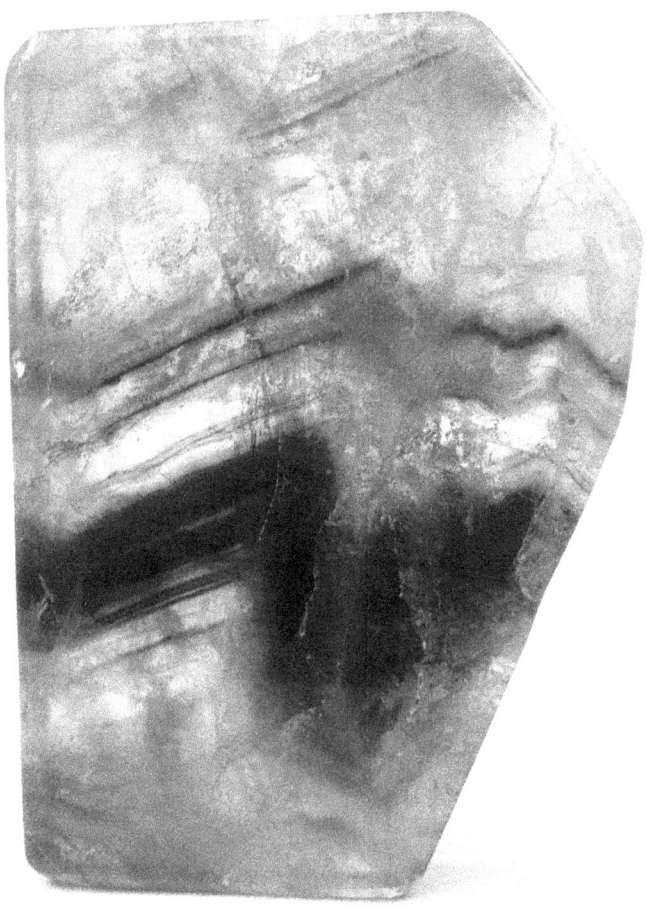

Green Aventurine

Crystal System: Trigonal
Astrological: Aries
Chakra: Heart, Spleen
Element: Air
Planet: Mercury
Hardness: 7
Composition: SiO_2 – Silicon Dioxide
Common Sources: Brazil, India, China, Italy, Russia, Tibet, Nepal

Healing
- Good for muscles, lungs, heart, adrenal glands, spleen, pituitary gland, urogenital system
- Relieving Anxiety and fear - Pre-exam and exam stress
- Protects, calms and soothes emotions.
- Aids relaxation
- Balancing male/female energies
- Enhances prosperity, leadership, decisiveness, compassion, empathy

Magical
- Prevents 'energy vampires' zapping energy
- Aids contact and channeling spirit guides
- Assists with ascertaining what makes you happy or unhappy
- Builds positive attitudes
- Increase perception
- 'good luck' stone

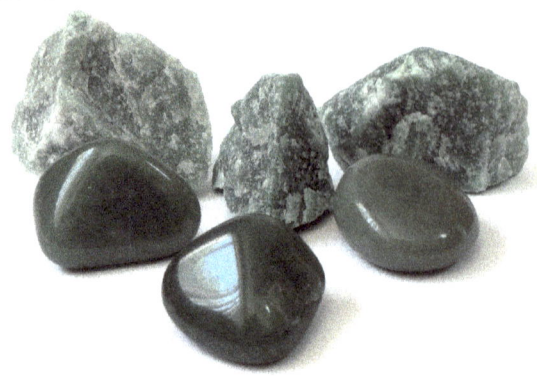

Hematite

Crystal System: Hexagonal
Astrological: Aquarius, Aries
Chakra: Earth, Root
Element: Fire
Planet: Saturn
Hardness: 5.5 – 6.5
Composition: Fe_2O_3 - Iron Oxide
Common Sources: USA, Canada, Italy, Brazil, Switzerland, Sweden, Venezuela, England

Healing
- Personal magnetism, brings strength, love, courage
- Aids mental processes, thought, memory, dexterity
- Assist in working with numbers/math
- Assists in coming to terms with mistakes as learning experiences.
- Boosts memory
- Helps with resistance to stress and to release stress

Magical
- Grounding stone, removes excess energy
- Support those with karmic battle in present life
- Can heal anger and hurt of warriors in previous life
- When worn on the right in right-handed people it can shut down metaphysical awareness
- Protects the Soul and guides it back into body during out-of-body experiences.
- Helps face shadow side of personality
- Repel and dissolve negativity

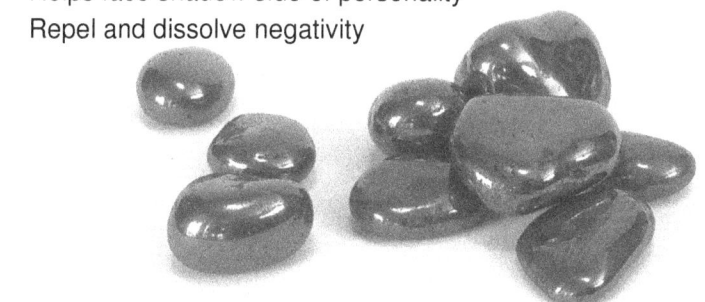

Herkimer Diamond

Crystal System: Trigonal
Astrological: Sagittarius
Chakra: Crown, Third Eye, purifies all
Element: Fire and Water
Planet: Sun
Hardness: 7
Composition: SiO2 – Silicon Dioxide
Source: Herkimer County, New York State, USA

Similar to clear quartz yet more potent.

Healing
- Reduces stress, fear and tension
- Strengthens metabolism and genetics
- Assists in removal of toxins
- May protect from radiation
- Encourages spontaneity
- Enhances memory
- Aids new beginnings
- Aids relaxation
- Being in the moment

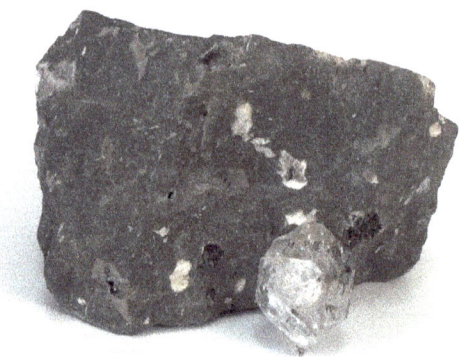

Magical
- Enhances inner vision
- Psychic abilities
- Dream recall and vivid dreaming
- Attunes energies, people, places and deities
- Allows clearer channels for telepathy
- Opens communication with spiritual teachers and guides
- Not to be worn for long periods – will draw you into a dream world.
- Able to produce and maintain a smooth constant energy flow.
- Can be substituted for diamonds in magic

Honey (Golden) Calcite

Crystal System: Hexagonal
Astrological: Leo
Chakra: Solar Plexus, Crown
Element: Fire
Planet: Sun
Hardness: 3
Composition: $CaCO_3$ – Calcium carbonate with impurities
Common sources: USA, UK, Belgium, Czech Republic, Slovakia, Peru, Iceland, Romania, Brazil,

Healing
- Calms and balances energy
- Helps with aggression and belligerence
- Intensifies clarity of life and events
- Spontaneity, energizing
- Brings vitality and inspiration
- Facilitates emotional intelligence – has a positive effect if hope is lost
- Connection emotions with intellect

Magical
- Enhances meditation: deep state of relaxation and spirituality
- Links to the highest source of spiritual guidance

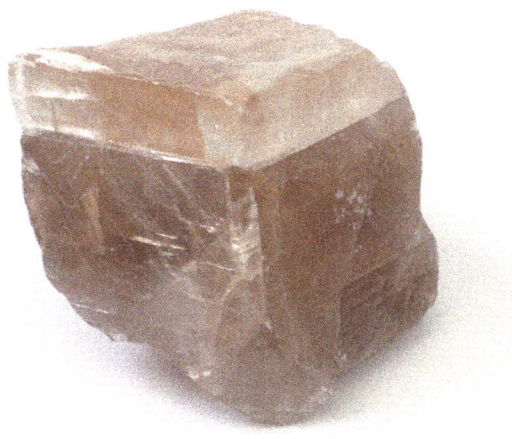

Iolite

Crystal System: Orthorhombic
Astrological: Aquarius, Taurus, Libra, Sagittarius
Chakra: Third eye, aligns all
Element: Water
Planet: Saturn
Hardness: 7
Composition: $Mg_2Al_4Si_5O_{18}$ Manesium aluminiun silicate
Common Sources: USA

Healing
- Good for submissiveness – strengthens self-confidence, taking charge of life
- Projects anti-martyr and anti-victim vibrations,
- Feeling comfortable in taking leadership role.
- Attracts friends and friendly help
- Flexibility in attitudes
- Balances male/female energies
- Inner strength
- Good for relationships
- Aids birthing problems / female problems
- Aids weight loss and detoxification
- Money management
- Living in the moment

Magical
- Moving thoughts into a higher realm
- Astral travel
- Shamanic visions and journeys
- Stimulates inner knowing
- Lessens emotional over-reactions
- Aura healing and clearing

♦ Assists in moving the thoughts into a higher realm
♦ Gives off an electrical charge that re-energizes the auric field and aligns aura

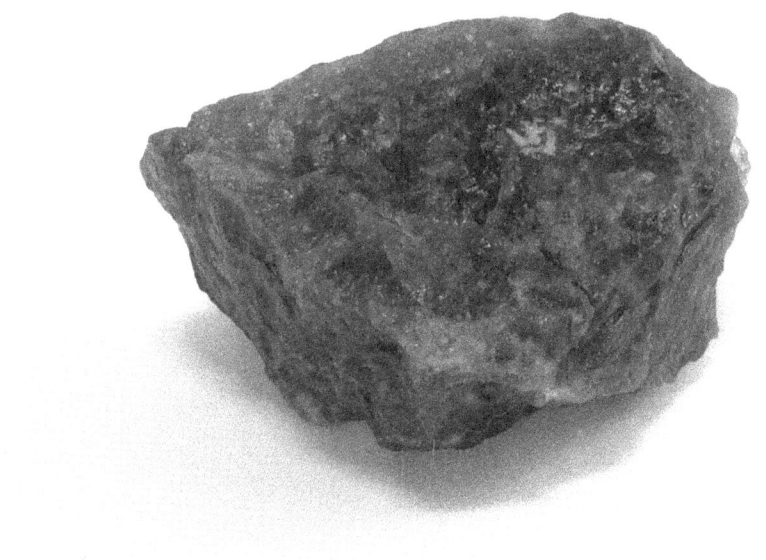

Kyanite

Crystal System: Triclinic
Astrological: Aries, Taurus, Libra
Chakra: Aligns all, Throat
Element:: Air and Water - Storm
Planet: Neptune
Hardness: 5.5-7
Composition: Al_2SiO_5 Aluminium silicate
Common Sources: USA, Brazil, Switzerland, Austria, Italy, India

AKA Disthene - Does not need cleansing

Healing
♦ Clears energetic field of person and creates a protective shield
♦ Excellent for attunement and meditation.
♦ Shows how current experience is connected to past behavior and choices
♦ Instills compassion
♦ Assists dream recall and promotes healing dreams.
♦ Helpful for making the transition through death
♦ Helps clear meridians. Restores Qi to the physical body
♦ Stabilizes biomagnetic field.
♦ Encourages speaking ones truth
♦ Cutting through fears, blockages, ignorance, illusion
♦ Opens spiritual and psychological truth

Magical
♦ Facilitates ascension process and spiritual maturation.
♦ Powerful transmitter and amplifier of high frequency energies
♦ Draws light body into physical realm
♦ Connects the higher mind to multi-dimensional frequencies
♦ Connection to guides
♦ The frequency of Kyanite directs you to act upon intuitive guidance

♦ Builds bridges between our inner and outer selves
♦ Helps to identify life-fulfilling vocation

Black Kyanite
♦ Powerful healing stone – keeps physical cells connected to the overall divine blueprint in order to maintain optimum health
♦ Assists in fully incarnating into this earth life
♦ Also moving back into the between life state to access current life plan and into other lives where necessary.
♦ Access potential future lives to view choices made in present.
♦ Assists those with the evolution of the earth

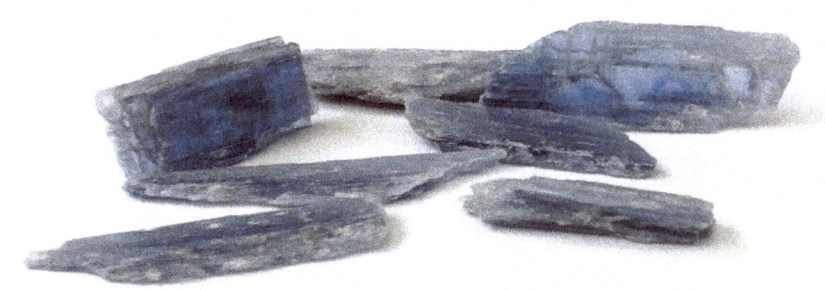

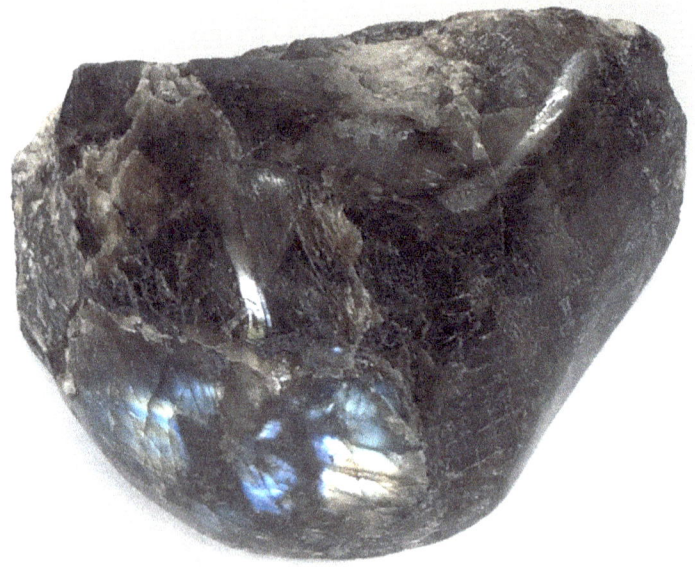

Labradorite

Crystal System: Triclinic
Astrological: Leo, Scorpio, Sagittarius
Chakra: Third eye, Crown,
Element: Water and Ice
Planet: Pluto
Hardness: 5-6.5
Composition: $(CaNa)(SiAl)_4O_8$ - Sodium calcium aluminosilicate
Common Sources: Italy, Greenland, Finland, Russia, Canada, Scandinavia

Healing
- Helps banish fears and insecurities and psychic debris from previous disappointments.
- Analysis and rationality are balanced with inner sight.
- Aids scientific analysis
- Stimulates willingness to get into action
- Opens subconscious mind to allow ideas to bubble up

Magical
- Transformation
- Prepares body and soul for the ascension process
- Highly mystical
- Protective stone raises consciousness
- Deflects unwanted energies from the aura
- Prevents energy leakage
- Holds esoteric knowledge – takes you into another world or into other lives
- Strengthens trust in the universe
- Removes projections and thought forms from other people that are hooked into the aura
- Enhances the energy flow between the aura and the chakras

Lapis Lazuli

Crystal System: Cubic
Astrological: Sagittarius
Chakra: Throat, Third eye, Crown
Element: Water
Planet: Saturn
Hardness: 5-6
Composition: $(NaCa)_8(AlSi)_{12}O_{24}S_2FeS$ $CaCO_3Al_2O_3$ – Sodium Calcium Aluminosilicate
Common Sources: USA, Chili, Italy, Middle East, Afghanistan, Russia

Healing
- Balances Female hormones – Menopause, PMS
- Immune, respiratory and nervous systems
- Enhances active listening and helps you to see and confront the truth
- Harmonizing conflict
- Aids in taking charge of your life
- Releases repressed anger
- Brings honesty, compassion and uprightness to the personality

Magical
- Ancient Egypt: believed to lead the soul into immortality and open the heart to love
- Key to spiritual attainment
- Enhances dream work and metaphysical abilities
- Stimulates personal and spiritual power
- Protective: alerting to psychic attack and returns the energy to its source. Reverse curses and disease caused by not speaking out
- Brings deep inner self-knowledge
- Powerful thought amplifier
- Bonding stone in love and friendship
- Used in ritual to attract spiritual love

Lepidolite

Crystal System: Monoclinic
Astrological: Libra
Chakra: All
Element: Water
Planet: Jupiter, Neptune
Hardness: 2.5-5
Composition: $AlSi_3O_{10}(OH,F)_2$ –Hydrated potassium aluminum silicate
Common Sources: USA, Czech Republic, Brazil, Madagascar, Dominican Republic

Healing
- Soothing to the nerves and relieves stress of everyday life
- Calming – soothes anger, hatred and other negative emotions.
- Promotes restful sleep – anti-nightmare
- Excellent for clearing electromagnetic pollution (place on computers or gird around house)

Magical
- Promotes and increases desire to seek spirituality
- Activating and opening all chakras
- Brings cosmic awareness
- Assists in shamanic or spiritual journeying, accessing Akashic records.
- Shows thoughts and feelings from other lives that are creating blockages in current life.
- Connectedness with the Whole.

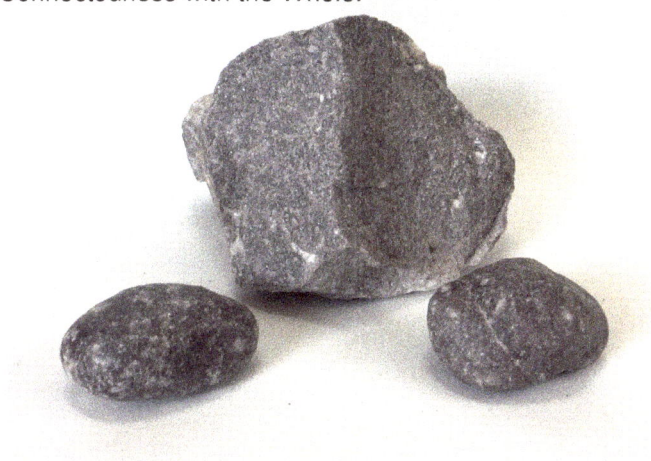

Malachite

Crystal System: Monoclinic
Astrological: Scorpio, Capricorn
Chakra: Heart, Solar plexus, Root, Sacral
Element: Earth
Planet: Venus
Hardness: 3.5-4
Composition: $Cu_2Co_3(OH)_2$ – Hydrous copper carbonate
Common Sources: USA, Australia, France, Russia, Germany, Zaire, Chile, Zambia, Romania, Congo, Middle East

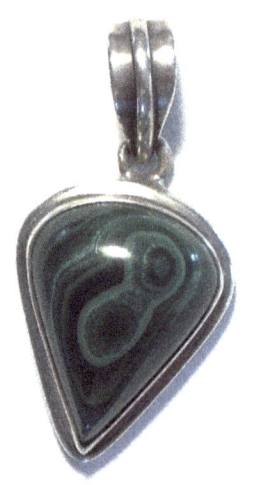

Healing
- Good for endurance
- Physical balance, eyesight, detoxing at a cellular level
- Eases birth
- Brings calm and emotional balance
- Releases past life and childhood trauma
- Energy conduit – has an intense influence
- Breaks unwanted ties
- Absorbs negative energies and pollutants from environment and body
- "Sleep Stone" – aids restful sleep

Magical
- Folklore: breaks into pieces to warn its wearer of forthcoming peril
- Protects against the evil eye, witchcraft, evil spirits
- Transformation
- Increases ability to send power towards magical goal
- Small pieces placed in each corner of a business or placed in cash register draws customers and money
- Good for dream interpretation and meditation
- Reflects the true character of person wearing – best not to wear when feeling negative

Moldavite

Crystal System: noncrystalline meteorite
Astrological: All
Chakra: All
Element: Fire
Planet: Uranus
Hardness: 5
Composition: extraterrestrial
Common Sources: Czechoslovakia, Bavaria, Moldavia

Healing
- Releases fixed ideas and outworn belief systems
- Opens the mind to new possibilities
- Promotes dreams and memories
- Promotes recognitions of spiritual origin

Magical
- Communication with higher self and with extraterrestrials
- Has its own cosmic connection, cosmic messengers
- Communication with Ascended Masters
- Facilitates Ascension
- Integrates divine blueprint and accelerates spiritual growth by downloading information from the Akashic Record. The information then has to be divinely processed before it is made conscious

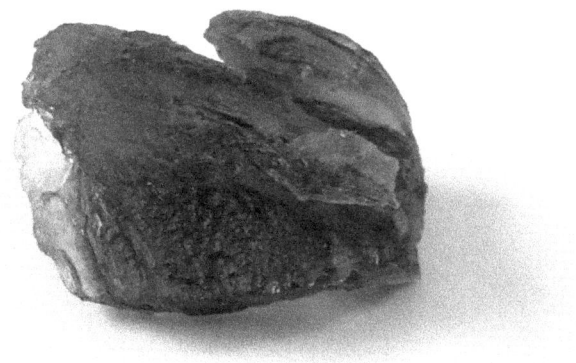

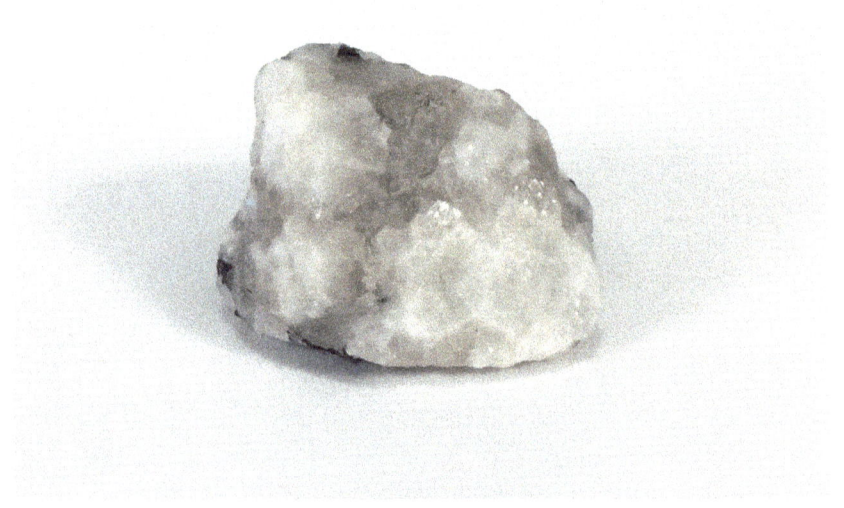

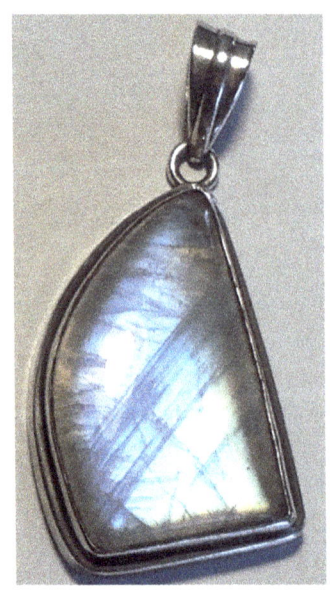

Moonstone

Crystal System: Monoclinic
Astrological: Cancer, Libra and Scorpio
Chakra: Heart
Element: Wind and Water
Planet: Moon
Hardness: 6
Composition: $K(AlSi_3O_8)$+Na, Fe, Ba – Potassium aluminium silicate
Common sources: India, Sri Lanka, Australia

Healing
- Helps with female reproductive system and childbirth. Reduces fluid retention, PMT, balancing hormones, menstruation
- Balances emotions – reduces over-reaction.
- Relieves stress and tension.
- Breaks up rigid attitudes and releases emotions
- Emotional ties to higher self.
- Helps see all possibilities and discard tunnel vision
- Health and prophecy, wisdom and passion
- Reducing stress and tension
- Brings calm, control, balance, confidence, composure, peace of mind. Helps with oversensitivity, pessimism,

Magical
- Connection to feminine side and Goddess
- Reveals truth behind illusions
- Enhances psychic perception and intuition
- Open gateway to subconscious (but only if ready)
- Communication with guides
- Understanding dreams
- Vulnerability
- Combats cycles/repeated patterns: new beginnings / endings

Obsidian

Crystal System: Amorphous
Astrological: Sagittarius
Chakra: Root
Element: Fire
Planet: Saturn
Hardness: 5-5.5
Composition: SiO_2 – Silicon Dioxide with impurities
Common Sources: Mexico, volcanic regions

Healing
- Exposes flaws, weaknesses, blockages, disempowering conditions
- Brings clarity to the mind and clears confusion
- Absorbs negative energies from the environment

Magical
- Flat surfaces used as scrying mirrors
- Has no boundaries or limitations – works extremely fast with great power
- Gives insight into the cause of disease
- Deep soul healing
- Helps heal festering emotions or trauma carried through from past lives
- Strongly protective – forms a shield against negativity, provides a grounding cord to base chakra to the Earths centre.
- Blocks psychic attach and negative spiritual influences
- Obsidian wand facilitates release of negative energies within the emotional body and protects the aura.
- Use to draw in aura more tightly in order to regroup scattered energies

Tip: if Obsidian works too powerfully, remove immediately and rebalance with Selenite and Rose Quartz

Snowflake Obsidian
- ♦ Stone of Purity
- ♦ Provides balance for body, mind and spirit
- ♦ Brings attention to ingrained patterns of behavior and gently releases emotional blockages.
- ♦ Teachers to surrender in meditation
- ♦ Isolation and loneliness become empowering with help from snowflake obsidian.

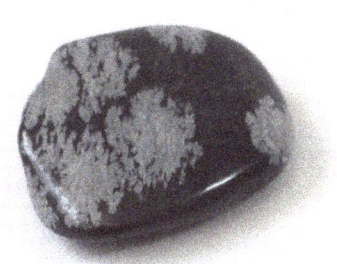

Mahogany Obsidian
- ♦ Earths, grounds and protects
- ♦ Strengthens aura
- ♦ Releasing energy blocks
- ♦ Balances polarities – light / dark, male / female
- ♦ Helps obtaining goals

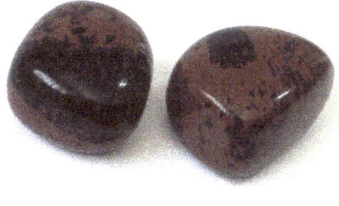

Rainbow Obsidian
- ♦ Transformation
- ♦ Assists with divination and scrying
- ♦ Attracts joy, abundance and prosperity
- ♦ Absorbs negative energies

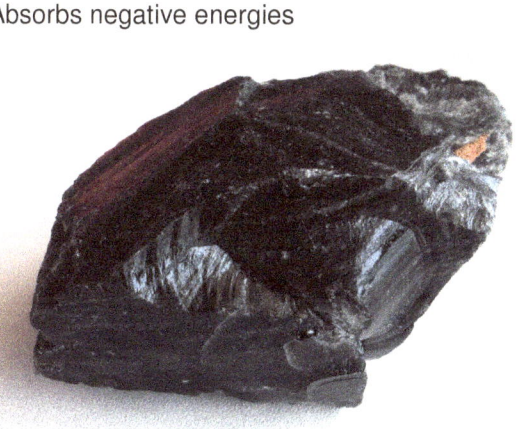

Phantom Quartz

Crystal System: Hexagonal
Astrological: All
Chakra: Soul Star, Heart, Crown
Element: Water
Planet: Moon
Hardness:7
Composition: SiO_2 – Silicon Dioxide
Common Sources: Brazil, Madagascar, USA

Healing
- Excellent for children to learn meditation, works well on children's illnesses, or adult's illnesses stemming from childhood.
- Great transition
- Releases stress
- Good for emotional clearing and the inner-self.
- Understanding and dealing with grief and loss

Magical
- Shamanic stone – tracing past lives and times of great transition
- Intensifies psychic awareness.
- Protects and shields whilst stimulating creativity and growth
- Helps to see hidden answers.

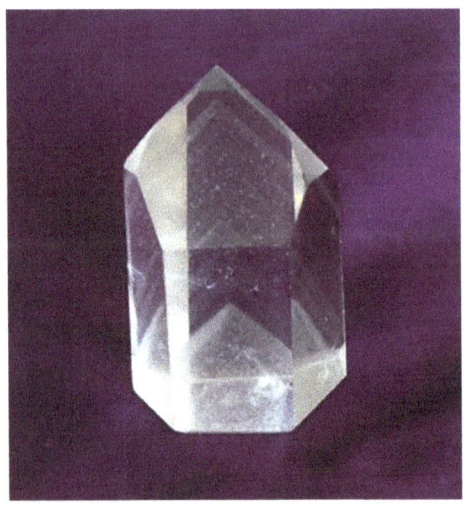

Red Jasper

Crystal System: Trigonal
Astrological: Aries, Scorpio
Chakra: Base, Sacral
Element: Fire
Planet: Mars
Hardness: 7
Composition: SiO_2 + Fe, O – Silicon dioxide with impurities
Common Sources: Worldwide

Healing
- Supreme Nurturer
- Sustains and supports during times of stress
- Unifies all aspect of life
- Balances yin and yang
- Aligns physical, emotional and mental bodies with the etheric realm
- Encourages honesty with oneself
- Aids quick thinking, organization and seeing projects through
- Transforms ideas into action
- Calm emotions
- Calms sexual aggressiveness and promotes sexual compatibility
- Assists in neutralizing electromagnetic and environmental pollution

Magical
- Facilitates shamanic journeying.
- Assists dowsing
- Aids dream recall
- Provides protection – absorbs negative energy and returns it to its source, is said to help protect against physical threats and psychic attack

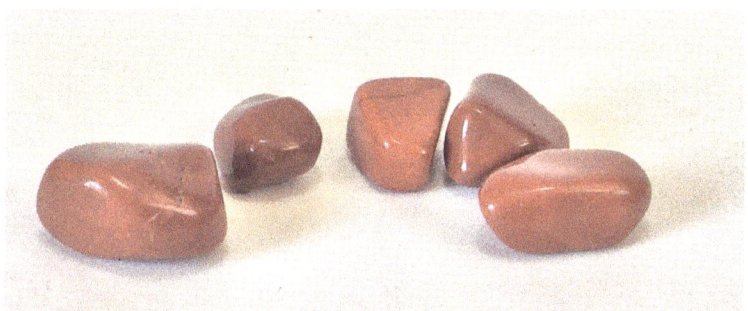

Rose Quartz

Crystal System: Trigonal
Astrological: Taurus and Libra
Chakra: Heart
Element: Water
Planet: Venus
Hardness: 7
Composition: SiO_2 – Silicon Dioxide with impurities
Common Sources: USA, Brazil, South Africa, Madagascar, Germany, India, Japan

Healing
- Clearing negative emotions – fear, anger, grief, guilt, jealousy, resentment
- Enhances compassion, forgiveness and unconditional love – especially for oneself
- Break up blockages in chakras caused by negative emotions
- Abuse recovery / Sexual Abuse recovery
- Balances sex drive and helps sexual frustration
- Helps build low self esteem - Anorexia / Bulimia
- To give and receive love
- Excellent for children – balancing temper tantrums and emotions and enhancing childhood experiences
- Improves circulation, kidney and adrenal function
- Opens the heart chakra
- Increase fertility, balances female reproductive system
- Calming, soothing, warmth and security
- Enhances female energy and qualities

Magical
- Aids communication with spirit guides
- Aura healing and clearing
- To attract romance, love and friendship

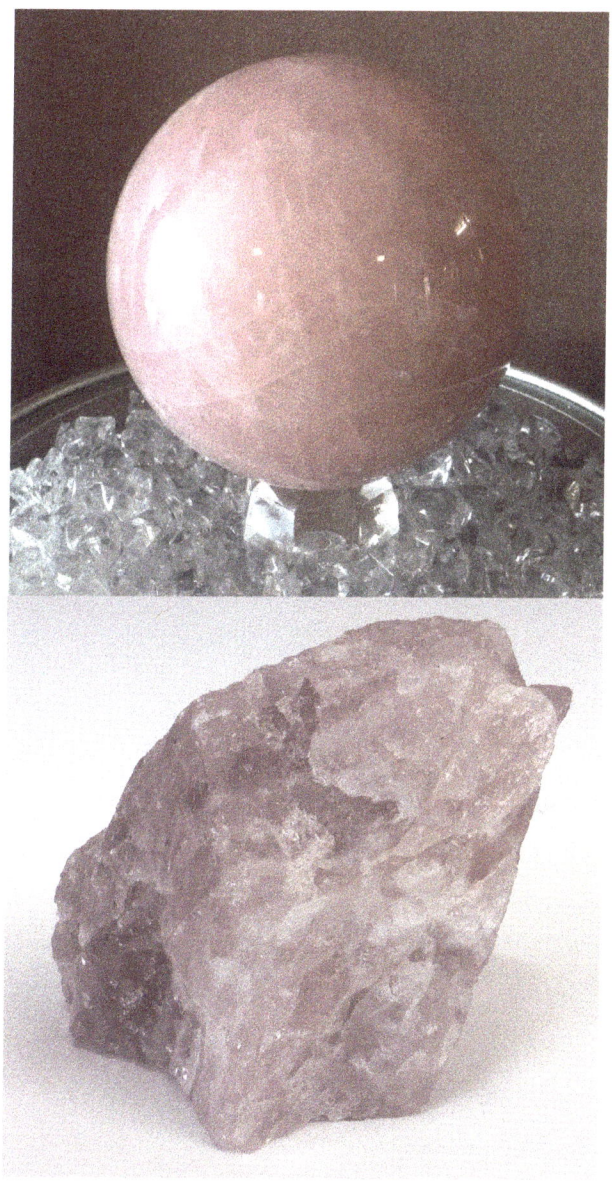

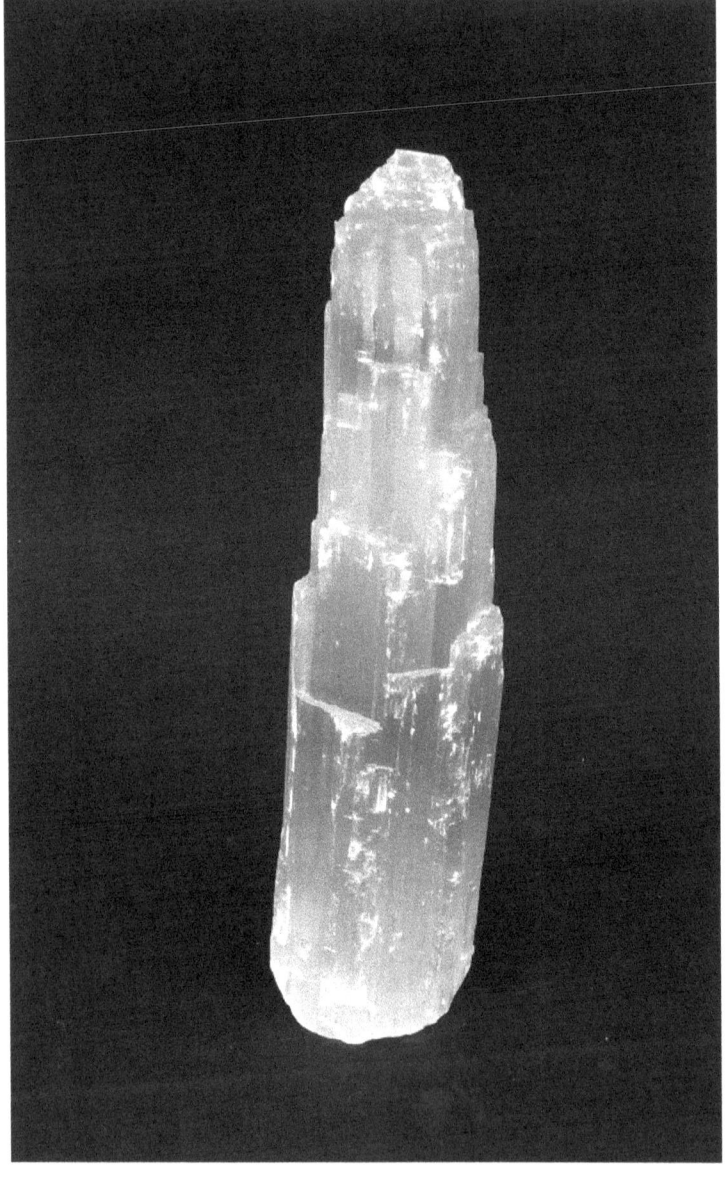

Selenite

Crystal System: Monoclinic
Astrological: Cancer, Taurus
Chakra: Soul Star, Higher Crown
Element: Water
Planet: Moon
Hardness: 2
Composition: $CaSO_{4-2}(H_2O)$ Hydrated calcium sulfate
Common Sources: England, USA, Mexico, Russia, Austria, Greece, Poland, Germany, France, Sicily

Healing
- Clarity and efficiency of mind
- Stabilizes and disperses erratic emotions
- Used to grid the home – ensures a peaceful atmosphere
- Lends energy to the body
- Exchange between lovers for reconciliation
- Enhances libido, fertility, regulates menstrual cycle
- Helps with abuse

Magical
- Access Angelic consciousness.
- Anchors light body in Earth vibration
- Can be used for scrying, to see the future or to ascertain what has occurred in the past
- Stabilizes and disperses erratic emotions.
- Selenite wands have a very pure vibration and can be used to detach entities or thought forms from the aura and preventing external influences on the mind.

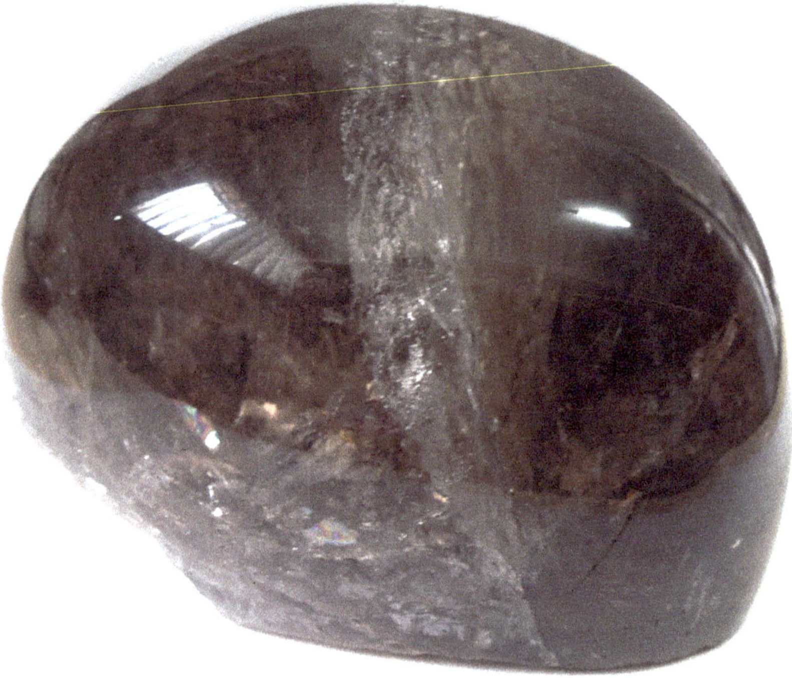

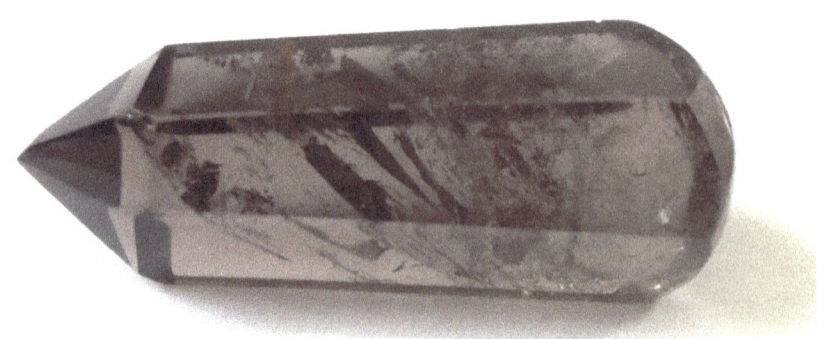

Smokey Quartz

Crystal System: Trigonal
Astrological: Capricorn, Sagittarius, Scorpio
Chakra: Root
Element: Earth
Planet: Earth
Hardness: 7
Composition: SiO_2 – Silicon Dioxide with lithium and aluminium
Common Sources: Worldwide

Healing
- Excellent for meditation – grounds and centers.
- Balance sexual energy
- Concentration
- Overcoming Depression and suicidal tendencies, severe mood swings
- Decreases fatigue and improves stamina, supports kidneys and adrenal glands
- Feet
- Fertility (energy block)
- Sedative and Relaxing
- Breaks up and releases subconscious blocks and negativity.
- Removing emotional blockages and the energies they attract : force you to look at past lives that are impacting the present – not only bringing to surface, but dissolving them

Magical
- Transmutes negative energy into positive - neutraliser Astral Travel – to ground
- Strengthens dream awareness and channeling – balances, grounds and protects
- Absorbs negativity from the aura and blocks psychic attack
- Linking with the Earth and its energies and nature spirits

Sodalite

Crystal System: Cubic
Astrological: Sagittarius
Chakra: Third Eye, Throat
Element: Water and Wind
Planet: Venus
Hardness: 5.5-6
Composition: $Na_4Al_3(SiO_4)_3$ – Sodium aluminium silicate chloride
Common Sources: USA, Canada, Brazil, France, Italy, Romania, Russia, Greenland.

Healing
- Face reality, release the past, and set goals for future.
- Clear out old mental patterns from subconscious
- Wisdom, Ideas, creative expression
- Enhances communication, creativity and sensuality
- Removing toxins that cause allergies
- Clears toxins, protects from pollutants
- Calming and clearing the mind - helps with confusion, inadequacy, mental unrest, oversensitivity, fear
- Reduces stress
- Improves physical endurance and perseverance
- Creativity
- Detoxification and Metabolism
- Balances the endocrine system and strengthens metabolism
- Balances male and female polarities

Magical
- Inner harmony - eases conflicts between conscious and subconscious minds
- Widens perspective
- Grounds and cuts through illusion
- Opens third eye and brings in inner psychic sight and intuitive knowledge

♦ Used for psychic development and mediation (especially if used with Lapis Lazuli and/or clear quartz)

Similar to Lapis Lazuli but milder – can be amplified by using other blue stones

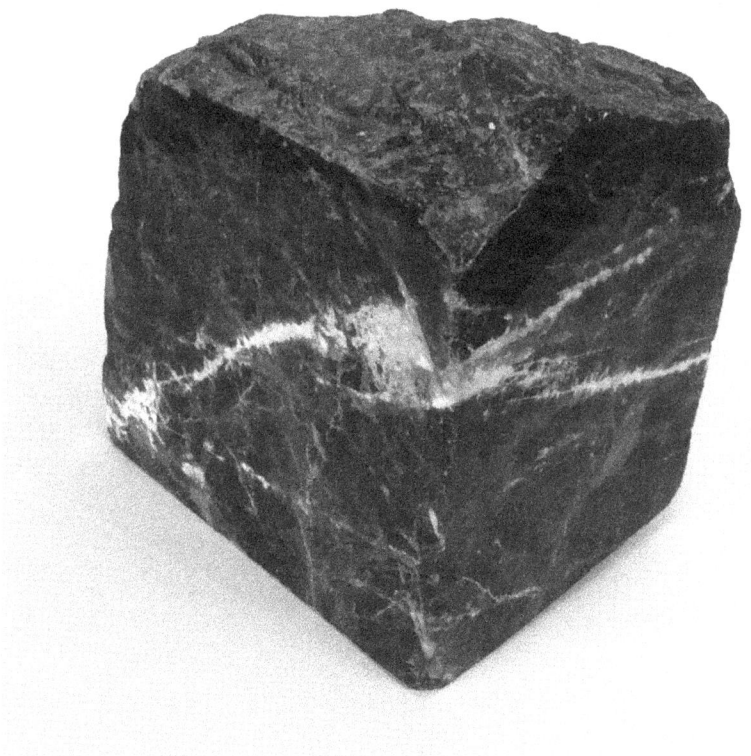

Tiger Eye

Crystal System: Trigonal
Astrological: Leo, Capricorn
Chakra: Third Eye, Sacral
Element: Fire
Planet: Sun
Hardness: 4-7
Composition: $NaFe_{+3}\{SiO_3\}_2$ Silicon dioxide with impurities
Common Sources: USA, Mexico, India, Australia, South Africa

Healing
- Helps with metal conditions such as personality disorders, issues of self-worth, self-criticism, blocked creativity
- Helps people who are 'spaced out' and uncommitted
- Emotional balancer
- Balances male/female energies
- Facilitates assertion and anchors change in the physical body
- Grounds and centers, strengthens connection of will and personal power.
- Helps recognize talents and overcoming faults.
- Supports an addictive personality in making changes)
- Beneficial for the weak and/or sick

Magical
- Protective Stone – Roman soldiers used to wear an engraved tigers eye to protect them in battle
- Draws spiritual energies to earth – combines earth energy with sun energy
- Assists correct use of Power – supports integrity and accomplishing goals.
- Used to promote wealth and money
- Strengthens convictions and confidence
- Strengthens courage

- Promotes energy flow through the body
- Used to delve into past lives and karmic ties
- Enhances psychic ability

*asbestos fibres

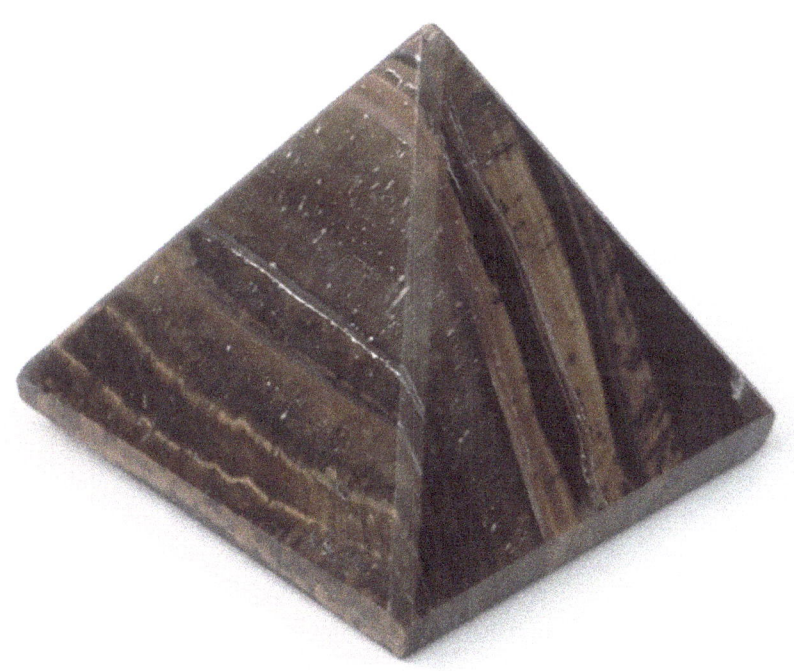

Yellow Jade

Crystal System: Complex
Astrological: Aries, Gemini and Libra
Chakra: Naval
Element: Fire and Water – Storm
Planet: Venus
Hardness: 6
Composition: $Na(AlFe)Si_2O_6$
Common sources: USA, Italy, China, Russia, Middle East, Myanmar

Healing
- Attracts courage and justice and wisdom
- Divine, unconditional love.
- Peaceful and nurturing
- Increases fertility
- Balance
- Strengthens heart, kidneys and immune system by cleansing the blood. Helps with poor digestion
- Energetic and stimulating with a contentment that brings Joy and happiness
- Helps understand the opposite sex
- A protector against danger for children

Magical
- Soul learnings
- Attracts master teachings through dreams – spiritual teachers
- Teaches interconnectedness of all beings
- Helps solve problems through your dreams
- Helps to recognize yourself as a spiritual being on a human journey

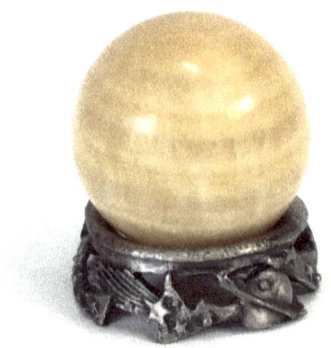

Ways of using and working with Crystals

Grids

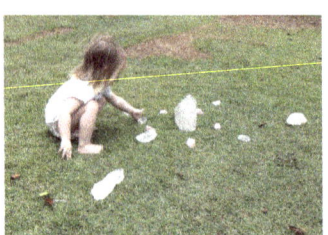

A crystal grid is geometric pattern of energetically aligned stones charged by intention, set in a sacred space for the purpose of focusing the Universal Life Force in order to manifest a particular object or for a particular purpose.

Crystal grids are an incredibly powerful energy tool to use when manifesting your desires, goals and intentions. So what is the difference between using individual stones versus a crystal grid? The power of a crystal grid comes from the union of energies created between the healing stones, sacred geometry and your intention. The combination of the power of crystals in a geometric pattern greatly strengthens your focused intention to manifest results much quicker.
The first step is to decide whether you will intuitively place the stones in a pattern (children are really good at this) or which geometric grid template you will need to use: hexagonal, spiral, 5-pointed star, infinity, flower of life, square. Each geometric shape has a different purpose.

Hexagonal (Star of David): attract/enhance romantic love, find a job, protection.
Spiral: Honouring Mother Earth, expansion.
5-pointed star: Calm and serenity, banish anxiety, protection.
Lemniscates (Infinity symbol): Abundance and prosperity, self love.
Flower of life: Good health, connection to Spirit.
Circle: Relationship enhancer, happiness and joy.
Square: Self protection, neutralizing negativity, stability.

NB Whilst a spiral grid may not usually be used for prosperity, it is used for expansion, so combining a spiral grid with prosperity crystals and intent, it can work to expand and increase finances.

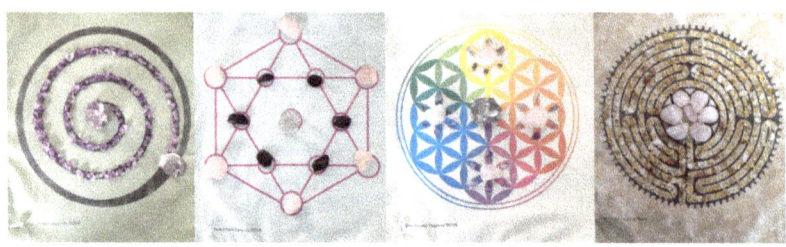

How to Make Your Crystal Grid:
Create your sacred space by burning a sage smudge stick to cleanse the energy of your space.
Visualize or write your intention on a piece of paper, place where the center of your crystal grid will be. Breathe deeply and state your intention aloud, or visualize it in your mind.

Setting out the grid:
Set your centre crystal as your focus piece, then start placing crystals from the centre and working your way out. As you are placing each stone into your crystal grid, make sure you keep your intention in mind. Then it's time to activate it.

Other things to consider when making a crystal grid
Do you want to align it with magnetic north (in northern hemisphere) or south (southern hemisphere). You can add candles, other healing crystals and energy tools around your crystal grid as well. Adding a mirror or magnifying glass can help reflect or magnify the intention. As will using an outer grid to amplify a power boost to the inner grid (i.e. working 2 grids in 1).

Now it's time to activate it. Take a quartz crystal point (can be small or large), wand or any crystal you are using as an activating crystal, and starting from the outside working inwards (unless it's a spiral geometric shape used for growth, then start in the middle and expand outwards), draw an invisible line between each stone to energetically connect each to the next (like dot to dots). You can recite an incantation, chant or repeatedly saying your intention whilst doing this to help keep the focus and raise energy whilst energetically connecting the crystals.

Once finished, re-affirm your intention once more and see it take form in your mind's eye - fully believing it to be true.
Maintenance: Grid should be left in place until you feel the grid has completed its task. This may be a few hours, a few days, a few weeks or months. If crystals become displaced (children, pets) then a full re-activation will be required. If in place for an extended period of time, monthly re-activation will be required to revitalize the intention and give it an energy boost.

Messages from the crystals

Choose a crystal to work with

Sit and meditate with the stone. Ask the crystal for a message to help with your question. Thank the crystal after you receive your message.

Example:
Rose quartz, I wish to receive more love in my life. Can you please show and tell me loud and clearly how can I receive this in my life now.

Citrine, I wish to receive more abundance in my life. Can you please show and tell me loud and clearly how can I receive this abundance now

Green Aventurine, I wish to receive more happiness in my life. Can you please show and tell me loud and clearly how can I receive this happiness now)

Malachite, I wish to receive more success in my business life. Can you please show and tell me loud and clearly how can I receive this success now

Amethyst, I wish to improve my psychic awareness in life. Can you please show and tell me loud and clearly how can I receive this psychic awareness now

Thank you, [crystal], for that beautiful message. I will certainly follow through with your helpful guidance.

Environment – windows, doorways, beds, TV's, electrical equipment, garden

- After smudging house/rooms, place crystals above doorways and windows to help prevent negative energies from re-entering.
- Placing crystals under your mattress can aid sleep, help with dream recall, assist in astral travelling. If worried about psychic attack or other negative energies whilst sleeping, sleep within a crystal grid which can be set up under bed or between the base and mattress.
- Himalayan salt lamps are beneficial for transmuting positive ion into negative ions (positive ions increase allergies etc)
- Placing next to plants to help them grow. Choosing green crystal can stimulate leaf, flower and fruit growth, black crystals help to ground and develop root growth. Rose Quartz infuses love into your plants to help them grow and Clear Quartz will help strengthen the plant
- Placing crystals on a window sill brings more energy and light into the room.
- Placing around electrical equipment helps to counter the effect of EMF's

Electromagnetic Fields (EMF's)
An electromagnetic field is the space around any electronic or magnetic device, where it has an active effect on it's surroundings. Electromagnetic pollution is the radiation given off by the electronics or magnets.

The effect EMF's have on our body
Our nervous system is constantly sending electrical signals to our brain – which is like a power station. Electrical signals are being sent through our nerves, blood vessels, cell membranes, myelin sheaths and muscles, we have bioelectrical closed circuits all of which are sending and receiving electrical messages. These are affected by external electromagnetic fields, which can be through areas of high natural geomagnetism or be seen in 'sick building syndrome', radio frequency hotspots etc. this can lead to enhanced electro sensitivity (it is essential to consult with a building biologist if this is the case)

Electro sensitivity can be seen with people who, when they touch electrical equipment computers will crash, radios will crackle, TV's will change station when they pass by. Some people will cause watches to run fast, run slowly or stop all together. When they touch people or animals they give electric shocks.

Symptoms of Electro stress
Feelings of pressure at the top and back of heads, sensation of crackling, worms or ants moving on their heads, headaches, cardiac rhythm disturbances - tachycardia, tinnitus, sudden mood changes. Neuro-transmitters in the brain effected (melatonin and serotonin) can be suddenly accelerated or depressed which effects mood, sleep, attention and memory.

Crystals that help counter the effects of EMF's include: clear quartz, amazonite, aventurine, black tourmaline, herkimer, unakite, diamond, lepidolite shungite, jasper

Gem Waters / Essences

Most people have heard of "Rescue Remedy" by Bach Flower Essences or "Emergency Essence" by Australian Bush Flower Essences. Essences are 'informed' by water, so flower essences are water informed by flowers, but what if you aren't a 'flower' person? I never resonated with flower essences, I am definitely a crystal person, but there wasn't any commercial crystal essences on the market that I could find – that's when I created "Debs Crystal Essence". There are currently 13 crystal essences in the range.

Gems waters can be used for drinking, healing, applying externally, bathing in. The water can be used in the garden to help plants grow, also to help with transplanting shock.

Caution: some crystals are extremely toxic and should not be used to make gem waters.

How to make:
- Placing directly in the water (be aware some crystals are toxic and tumbled stones can covered in lacquer)
- Test tube method – placing the crystal in a test tube which is then placed in a glass of water (the crystal does not actually touch the water).
- Glass of water on a crystal slab
- Transferring energy from crystal by placing the crystal next to the glass

Pendants / Jewelery

Worn on a long chain around the neck so that it covers the heart chakra – stimulates the thymus, increases immune system function. Amplifies the body's energies and creates protection from negative energies.

Worn on choker or short chain around neck – stimulates thyroid and parathyroid, excellent for sore throats and respiratory problems. Excellent for communication.

Worn around the wrist as a bracelet. – left wrist will work with the crystal energies as a receiver of their energy – it will bring it into your energy system and chakras to be used in a harmonious way to restore balance to your bodies. It is also energizing and revitalizing. Worn on the right side helps clear old traumas, patterns pain and blocks. It can draw out and release toxins on physical, etheric, emotional, mental and spiritual levels.

Worn around the ankle – the left side is more beneficial for grounding, being in the body and nurturing. Connect to the Earth and receiving the earth's energy and the connectedness of all. On the right ankle helps ground your purpose – walking your path with confidence and ease. Standing strong in your own light.

Healing / Chakra Balancing

"Psychoenergy centres, where the subtle body meets the physical body"
Peter Sherwood

"Vortexes of psychic energy through which the life force is channelled in the human body, mind and spirit………..Chakras control the flow of energy to and from the aura"
Cassandra Eason

- Spin in a clockwise direction when open. Funnel / cone shaped
- Associated herbs - Not to be ingested, but rather they are energetically compatible

Root
- Name: Muladhara
- Location – Base of spine
- Sound – Lam
- Element / Gland / Area of Body / Metaphysical
  ◇ Earth; Adrenals; Spinal column, kidneys; Grounding, connection to our roots/past, kundalini energy
- Colour – Red
- Imbalances
  ◇ pain/tension in legs, feet, skeleton (including teeth), large intestines, fear, anxiety
- Herbs
  ◇ basil, comfrey, horsestail
- Crystal associations
  ◇ Ruby, Garnet, Black Tourmaline, Red Jasper, Rhodonite, Smoky Quartz, Obsidian, Hematite, Bloodstone, Lodestone, Jet

Sacral
- Name: Svadishthana
- Location - below navel – womb in women
- Sound – Vam
  Element / Gland / Area of Body / Metaphysical
  ◇ Water; Gonads; Reproductive organs; Desires, sexuality
- Colour – Orange

- ♦ Imbalance
  - ◇ Seek emotional satisfaction through eating disorders, smoking, drug and alcohol abuse
- ♦ Herbs
  - ◇ freesia, gardenia, lemon balm, poppy, wintergreen
- ♦ Crystal associations
  - ◇ Dark Citrine, Carnelian, Orange Calcite, Amber

Solar plexus
- ♦ Name: Manipura
- ♦ Location - between navel and sternum
- ♦ Sound - Ram
- ♦ Element / Gland / Area of Body / Metaphysical
  - ◇ Fire; Pancreas; Stomach, liver, gallbladder, nervous system; Personal power, individuality, 'gut feeling'
- ♦ Colour – Yellow
- ♦ Imbalance
  - ◇ Digestive disorders, hyperactivity, lack of self-confidence, obsessions, inability to empathise
- ♦ Herbs
  - ◇ Allspice, basil, coriander, ginger, peppermint, tarragon
- ♦ Crystal associations
  - ◇ Citrine, Gold, Pyrite, Tiger Eye, Amertrine, Amber

Heart
- ♦ Name: Anahata
- ♦ Location - Centre of chest i.e. sternum
- ♦ Sound - Yam
- ♦ Element / Gland / Area of Body / Metaphysical
  - ◇ Air; Thymus; Heart, Blood, Circulatory system; Emotions and healing, self love, spiritual love, awareness of past lives and other worlds
- ♦ Colour – Green/Pink
- ♦ Imbalances
  - ◇ Breathing difficulties, allergies, oversensitivity to emotions, inability to feel emotions

- ♦ Herbs
  - ◇ Echinacea, feverfew, heather, mugwort, pennyroyal, thyme, verbena, yarrow
- ♦ Crystal associations
  - ◇ Emerald, Malachite, Rose Quartz, Dioptase, Apatite, Sapphire, Jade, Amazonite, Turquoise, Smithsonite, Aquamarine, Aventurine, Chryoprase, Peridot, Green Tourmaline, Pink Tourmaline, Kunzite, Moonstone, Phantom Quartz

Throat

- ♦ Name: Vishudda
- ♦ Location - Throat
- ♦ Sound - Ham
- ♦ Element / Gland / Area of Body / Metaphysical
  - ◇ Sound; Thyroid; Bronchial and vocal apparatus, lungs; Self expression
- ♦ Colour – Blue
- ♦ Imbalances
  - ◇ sore throats, swollen glands in the neck, mouth ulcers, confusion
- ♦ Herbs
  - ◇ Dill, lemon verbena, lily of the valley, parsley, peppermint
- ♦ Crystal associations
  - ◇ Blue Lace Agate, Sapphire, Sodalite, Lapis Lazuli, Blue Topaz, Celestite, Angelite, Aquamarine, Turquoise, Chrysocolla, Amazonite

Third eye

- ♦ Name: Anja
- ♦ Location - in between eyes/eyebrows
- ♦ Sound - Om
- ♦ Element / Gland / Area of Body / Metaphysical
  - ◇ Light; Pituitary; Lower brain, left eye, ears, nose, nervous system; Intuitive insight, psychic functioning and clear-seeing

- ♦ Colour – Indigo
- ♦ Imbalances
  - ◇ Ear aches, blurred vision without reason, headaches, migraines, blocked sinuses, insomnia, nightmares
- ♦ Herbs
  - ◇ Borage, cinquefoil, coltsfoot, hyssop
- ♦ Crystal associations
  - ◇ Lapis Lazuli, Sapphire, Kyanite, Azurite, Tanzanite, Amethyst, Labradorite, Angelite, Sodalite

Crown

- ♦ Name: Sahasrara
- ♦ Location – crown/top of head
- ♦ Sound – Aum / Silence
- ♦ Element / Gland / Area of Body / Metaphysical
  - ◇ Spirit; Pineal; Upper brain, right eye; Wisdom
- ♦ Colour – Purple/Violet (White - all colours)
- ♦ Imbalances
  - ◇ Headaches, migraines, inefficient immune system, forgetfulness, sense of alienation from the world
- ♦ Herbs
  - ◇ Bay, chamomile, juniper, marigold, rosemary, St John's Wort
- ♦ Crystal associations
  - ◇ Amethyst, Sugilite, Lepidolite, Labradorite, Ametrine, Angel Aura Quartz, Angelite, Fluorite, Clear Quartz, Diamond, Phantom Quartz

A simple way to revitalize your energy. You can lie on your back with a crystal placed on each chakra. Or place crystals in a circle and sit in the middle.

Pendulum

A pendulum is a weight suspended by a thread or chain. Using a pendulum can be an easy way to learn divination, however, it is useful for asking yes/no questions only. First you need to establish a yes/no swing or oscillation. This can be done by asking a question you know the answer eg. Am I 40 years old?

If the crystal does not move when asking a question, this can be an indication that either you need to rephrase the question or you are not meant to know the answer at this time. It is also important to know who you are working with – which higher being. Is it your   Higher Self, an Angelic Being, Lords of Karma or somebody else.

Establish yes/no swing or oscillation

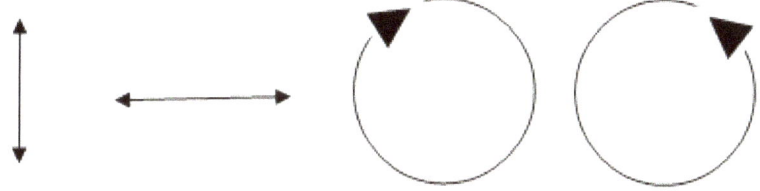

Tip: Something to be aware of: are you using receptive or projective hand – are you receiving information or influencing movement (see footnote 3 p 12).

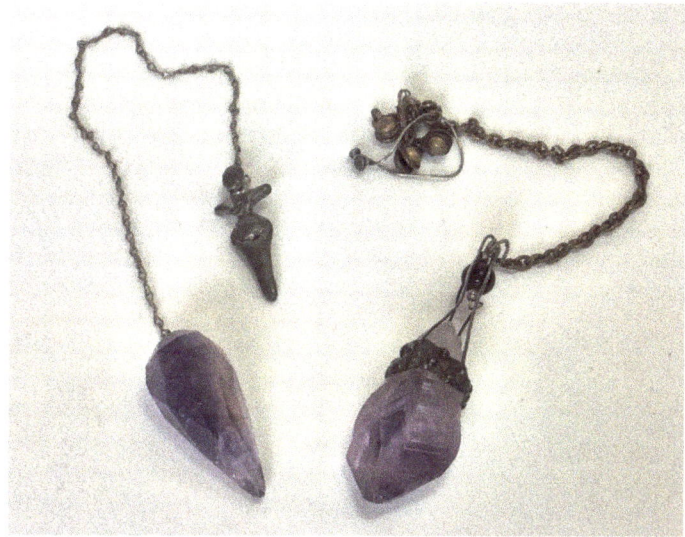

Correspondences

Crystals listed by crystal system

Hexagonal

Sapphire – pink, blue, yellow, green
Strawberry Quartz
Phantom Quartz
Aura Quartz – Rose, red, opal
Calcite – Mangano
Covellite
Cinnabar
Beryl
Heliodor (golden beryl)
Morganite (pink beryl)
Bixbite (red beryl)
Rhodochrosite
Zincite
Calcite – red, orange, green, blue
Icelandic Spar
Quartz – drusy, blue. Rutile, clear
Indicolite (blue tourmaline)
Emerald
Sugilite
Magnesite
Apatite – yellow
Aquamarine
Hematite
Dioptase

Cubic

Halite – Pink
Garnet
Cuprite
Fluorite
Spinel – Red, orange, blue
Lapis Lazuli
Sodalite
Boji Stone
Peacock Ore
Lodestone
Diamond
Pyrite

Trigonal

Rose Quartz
Amethyst
Smoky Quartz
Ametrine
Eudialyte
Carnelian – pink, orange
Pietersite
Sardonyx
Onyx
Jasper – red, brescciated, poppy, green, leopardskin, rainforest
Cinnabar jasper
Agate – pink, red, fire, tree, green, moss, dendritic, blue lace
Aventurine – peach, red, green, blue

Tourmaline – watermelon, pink, red (rubellite), yellow, green
Chalcedony – pink, red, blue
Ruby
Tiger's Eye – Red, golden, blue
Quartz – golden healer
Citrine
Mookaite
Herkimer – Enhydro, clear
Bloodstone (Heliotrope)
Chrysoprase – lemon, green
Smithsonite

Tetragonal
Tugtupite
Rutile
Wulfenite
Apophyllite
Zircon – red, orange

Orthorhombic
Danburite
Topaz – pink, blue
Zoisite – Pink (Thulite)
Sulfur
Peridot
Prehnite
Variscite
Nuummite
Shattuckite
Chrysocolla
Angelite
Celestite
Cat's Eye
Dumortierite
Stibnite
Anhydrite
Iolite

Tanzanite
Chiastolite (cross stone)
Argonite
Hemimorphite

Triclinic
Sunstone – pink
Rhodonite
Turquoise- Tibetan, standard
Amazonite
Ajoite
Kyanite
Larimar
Labradorite
Chrysanthemum stone

Monoclinic
Kunzite
Jade – red, orange, green
Muscovite
Unakite (epidote)
Desert Rose
Staurolite (fairy cross)
Selenite – peach
Serpentine – red, green.
Malachite
Lepidolite
Moonstone
Howlite- white, blue
Charoite
Diopside
Seraphinite
Chlorite
Fuchsite
Serpentine
Azurite

Amorphous
Opal – cherry, Ethiopian, fire, water

Obsidian – black, rainbow
Jet
Apache tear
Tektite

Complex
Atlantasite™
Quantum Quattro™
Eilat Stone
Tiger iron
Shiva Lingam

Crystal listed by Planet

Sun - Energy – physical and magical, ambition, business success, prosperity and abundance, legal matters, protection, masculine energy, healing, illumination.
- Amber
- Carnelian
- Citrine
- Clear Quartz
- Diamond
- Herkimer Diamond
- Golden Calcite
- Sunstone
- Tiger Eye
- Topaz
- Zircon

Mercury – self-improvement, studying, divination, communication, wisdom, strengthening mental agility.
- Agate
- Green Aventurine
- Jasper

Venus – love, fidelity, romance, friendship, pleasure, lust, joy and happiness, art, beauty
- Azurite
- Blue Calcite
- Blue Tourmaline

- Celestite
- Chrysocolla
- Chrysoprase
- Emerald
- Green Calcite
- Green Tourmaline
- Jade
- Kunzite
- Lapis Lazuli
- Malachite
- Peridot
- Pink Calcite
- Pink Tourmaline
- Rose Quartz
- Sodalite
- Turquoise
- Watermelon Tourmaline

Earth – peace, grounding and centering, stability, gardening
- Smoky Quartz
- Argonite

Moon - Love, peace, compassion, spirituality, fertility, feminine energy, enhancing psychic abilities – intuition and telepathy, the home, gardening, prophetic dreams, sleep
- Aquamarine
- Beryl
- Clear Quartz
- Phantom Quartz
- Moonstone
- Sapphire
- Selenite

Mars – raw power, physical strength, courage, aggression, destruction, overcoming rivalry, protection, self-defence, military success.
- Red Jasper
- Bloodstone
- Garnet

- Rhodocrosite
- Rhodonite
- Ruby

Jupiter – enhancing psychic ability, spirituality, meditation, idealism, expansion
- Amethyst
- Lepidolite
- Celestite
- Sugilite

Saturn – preservation, protection, stability, grounding, centering, purification
- Iolite
- Hematite
- Obsidian
- Lapis Lazuli
- Jet

Uranus – releases fixed ideas and outworn belief systems
- Moldavite

Neptune – accessing higher realms, spirituality
- Amethyst
- Fluorite
- Lepidolite
- Kyanite
- Celestite
- Turquoise

Pluto – free will, letting go and releasing, stripping away ego
- Black Tourmaline
- Labradorite
- Tourmalated Quartz

Bibliography

Ahsian N, 1997, *The Crystal Ally Cards: The Crystal Path to Self Knowledge*, Heaven and Earth Publishing, Marshfield, VT

Barralet A, 2014, *Crystal Connections*, Animal Dreaming Publishing, Lismore

Berkovitch S, 1996, *Crystal Guide*, Hihorse Publishing Pty Ltd, Glen Iris, Vic

Brennan, Barbara Ann, 1987, *Hands of Light*, Bantam Books, New York

Conway D.J., 1999, Crystal Enchantments: A complete guide to stones and their magical properties, The Crossing Press Inc, Freedom, CA

Cowan D, Arnold C, 2003, *Ley Lines and Earth Energies: A groundbreaking exploration of the Earths natural energy and how it effects our health*, Adventures Unlimited Press, Illinois USA

Cunningham S, 1999, *Cunningham's Encyclopedia of Crystal, Gem and Metal Magic*, Llewellyn Publications, St Paul, MN

Dunwich G, 2001, *Exploring Spellcraft: How to Create and Cast Effective Spells*, The Career Press Inc, New Jersey

Eason C, 2001, *Chakra Power*, Quantum, England

Eason C, 2003, t*he illustrated directory of healing crystals: a comprehensive guide to 150 crystals and gemstones*, Collins and Brown, London

Elsbeth M, 2002, *Crystal Medicine,* Llewellyn Publications, Minnesota

George M, 1999, *Crystals: Pocket Guide to natural Healing Powers Revised Edn*, In The Light Publishing, Laidley, Australia

George M, 2000, *Crystals: Pocket Guide to natural Healing Powers Vol 2*, In The Light Publishing, Laidley, Australia

Gienger M, 2005, *Healing Crystals: The A-Z Guide to 430 Gemstones*, Earthdancer Books, Scotland

Gienger M, Goebel J, 2009, *Gem Water*, Earthdancer Books, Scotland

Gillotte G, 2003, *Sacred Stones of the Goddess: Using Earth Energies for Magical Living*, Llewellyn Publications, Minnesota

Hall J, 2007, *The Encyclopedia of Crystals*, Octopus Publishing, London

Jones W, Jones B, 1997, *The Magic of Crystals*, Harper Collins Publishers, Sydney

King S, 1997, *Crystals: Gateways of Light and Unity*, Evenstar Creations, Kin Kin

Lilly S, 2001, *Crystal Decoder*, Quarto Publishing, London

Permutt P, 2007, *The Crystal Healer*, Cico Books, New York

Sabrina L, 2000, *Exploring Wicca: the beliefs, rites, and rituals of the Wiccan religion,* The Career Press Inc, New Jersey

Sherwood, Peter, 2005, *HEALING The History, Philosophy and Practice of Natural Medicine*, Australian College of Natural Medicine, Brisbane

Simmons R, Ahsian N, 2015, *The Book of Stones: Who They Are and What They Teach Revised Edn*, Heaven and Earth Publishing, East Montpelier VT USA

Simpson S, 1997, *The Book of Crystal Healing*, Gaia Books Ltd, London

Sonnenberg P, 2003, *The Great Pendulum Book*, Sterling Publishing Co. Inc., New York

Virtue, Doreen, 1998, *Chakra Clearing*, Hay House Inc, Sydney

http://www.crystalsrocksandgems.com/Crystal_Therapy_and_Healing/Wands.html viewed: February 2016

https://crystal-cure.com/article-wands-healing.html viewed: February 2016

www.hibiscusmooncrystalacademy.com viewed: February 2016

For workshop enquiries and information on obtaining additional copies of this book, crystal essences or crystal grid cloths.

Mail and email orders.
Wholesale enquiries.

Please contact:
Debra Cushing
RED RASPBERRY NATUROPATHICS
PO Box 5560
Alexandra Hills Qld 4161
Australia
deb@redraspberrynaturopathics.com.au
www.redraspberrynaturopathics.com.au

www.ingramcontent.com/pod-product-compliance
Lightning Source LLC
Chambersburg PA
CBHW040336300426
44113CB00021B/2762